HOW I CONQUERED BREAST CANCER WITHOUT CHEMOTHERAPY

My Journey From a Mess to a Message

Francisca Epale, MA, DTM

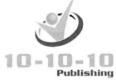

10-10-10
Publishing

May this book empower
& inspire you.
Happy reading
Francisca B. Epale

How I Conquered Breast Cancer Without Chemotherapy:
My Journey From a Mess to a Message
http://breastcancerconquerednow.com
Copyright © 2021 Francisca Epale

ISBN: 978-1-77277-445-0

References to internet websites (URLs) were accurate at the time of writing. Authors and the publishers are not responsible for URLs that may have expired or changed since the manuscript was prepared.

Limits of Liability and Disclaimer of Warranty
The author and publisher shall not be liable for your misuse of the enclosed material. This book is strictly for informational and educational purposes only.

Warning – Disclaimer
The purpose of this book is to educate and entertain. The author and/or publisher do not guarantee that anyone following these techniques, suggestions, tips, ideas, or strategies will become successful. The author and/or publisher shall have neither liability nor responsibility to anyone with respect to any loss or damage caused, or alleged to be caused, directly or indirectly by the information contained in this book.

Medical Disclaimer
This book details the author's personal experiences with and opinions about cancer, with a focus on breast cancer. The author is not a [or your] healthcare provider.

The medical or health information in this book is provided as an information resource only, and is not to be used or relied on for any diagnostic or treatment purposes. This information is not intended to be patient education, does not create any patient-physician relationship, and should not be used as a substitute for professional diagnosis and treatment.

Publisher
10-10-10 Publishing
Markham, ON   Canada

Printed in Canada and the United States of America

Note to the Reader:
Throughout the book, the names of the healthcare providers who worked with me have not been mentioned to ensure confidentiality and privacy.

Contents

I dedicate this book to my family members
who have passed away from different kinds of cancer.

Testimonials

If there is one book you need to read, it is this one. I have known Francisca for more than 10 years and I was very flattered, happy and pleased that she asked me to write a testimony for her fourth book *How I Conquered Breast Cancer Without Chemotherapy: My Journey from a Mess to a Message.*

One of my favorite chapters is chapter 9 which deals with the Power of Faith and Hope. She emphasizes that with God all things are possible. With her strong faith in God, through daily prayers, devotionals, intercessory prayers and Bible reading, they uplifted her spiritually which indirectly healed her physically to conquer one of the deadliest diseases in the world! Grab a copy to learn about preventive measures to heal cancer using unorthodox methods. This is a must read!!!

Pastor Lumembo Tshiswaka
Missionary to Ethiopia
Author of "I Want to See God" - A short play - 2020

I am happy to say that the award-winning book *How I Conquered Breast Cancer without Chemotherapy: My Journey from a Mess to a Message* is one of the most practical books I have read in a long time.

It is educational, entertaining, and inspirational. This book should be made available at women's conferences, churches, sororities, women's shelters, libraries, bookstores and to family members.

There is a lot to learn in this book such as intermittent fasting, square breathing and brushing your teeth with aluminum-free baking soda to name but a few!.

Keep up the good work, Francisca.

Jeffrey Ginsbarg
Retail Health Business Consultant

When I learnt that Francisca had written her fourth book, *How I Conquered Breast Cancer Without Chemotherapy: My Journey from a Mess to a Message,* I decided to find out what she has to share with the world.

Her writing leaves me wanting to dig deeper into the book to learn more about her personal healing journey. Francisca's healing journey steps from her motivation to end her family's cancer history where five members of her family succumbed to cancer. This book is not only an interesting and captivating read with humour, it is also very educational and insightful. Both men and women can benefit from this book's numerous interesting topics from holistic nutrition, necessary lifestyle changes, planting good seeds and more. I can't wait to get my copy and start implementing some of the strategies mentioned in the book to improve my very own health situation.

What are you waiting for? Grab a copy now.

Leah Xing
Office Worker

I have known the award-winning author Francisca Epale since elementary school. She was two classes behind me. I also knew some of her family members who passed away from cancer, so I totally appreciate, empathize and understand why she would write such a book. Francisca shares through a step-by-step formula the secret sauce she used to conquer her breast cancer without the use of traditional medicine. The book *How I Conquered Breast Cancer Without Chemotherapy: My Journey from a Mess to a Message* is one of a kind. It is a must-read to include in your library!

Thomas Eyambe, LL. B, DES
Former Director of General Affairs
Prime Ministers Office, Yaounde, Cameroon
Customs Expert, Licensed in the Central African Economic & Monetary Union

A very inspirational story to read. The insights are authentic and inspiring. There is a sense of balance in her well being that will truly empower others who are in similar journeys as Francisca! It's a must read and educational too. I am proud of her resilience!

Wilma David
International Alternative Healing
Practitioner & NLP Coach

The award-winning author, Francisca Epale is one of my regular attendees on my 15-minute daily sales motivational calls.

I highly recommend *How I Conquered Breast Cancer Without Chemotherapy: My Journey from a Mess to a Message* to everyone, regardless of their occupation.

Through the lens of a sales trainer and sales coach for more than 22 years, I find the book title very captivating, catchy, and thought-provoking. Statistics states that 1 in 8 women will be diagnosed with breast cancer in their life time. The author uses a magic bullet list of strategies to conquer her breast cancer such as holistic nutrition, self-care, the power of faith and more....

I highly endorse these strategies and would encourage you to buy several copies for your families, friends, team members, employees or staff. They will be eternally grateful to you for this awe-inspiring book!

Eric Lofholm
International Sales Trainer & Sales Coach
Author of *The System*

It is with profound joy and excitement that I am expressing how I feel about the award-winning book *How I Conquered Breast Cancer Without Chemotherapy: My Journey from a Mess to a Message.* This book is brilliantly written, with apt quotations to match the chapter headings. The fact that Francisca lost five family members to cancer is a strong testament to why she looked for alternate treatment for her breast cancer. As she mentioned in her book, cancer does not have to be a death sentence. There is light at the end of the tunnel.

Her honest ability to share her private healing journey with the world stands to be admired.

Trudy Bak
Real Estate Investor

Wow! What an honest and useful guide for acting to prevent cancer before a diagnosis or fight cancer after one. Francisca covers practical areas of your life that you can easily improve to improve your cancer odds, such as developing the right positive mindset for healing, daily practices to start, cleaning up your nutrition, environment, and the products you use in the bathroom, kitchen and for your home. She examines the impact of stress on cancer and so much more. This is a MUST READ if you already have cancer or would rather never have cancer in the first place. it is not a guarantee, but it is a solid and practical approach to preserving your health.

As someone who heard the words "Cervical Cancer" when I was 17, I can tell you I have lived my life very differently ever since. It feels empowering to know that I am doing all that I can to keep cancer out of my body now, and that includes building a happy life, with balance, organic food most of the time, alkaline water, low EMF exposure, managed stress and much more. I am also proof that cancer can be a new beginning, and not just the end as we fear. Please share this book with your loved ones, for as Francisca says "their life may depend on it."

Hailey Patry
Your True Happiness Coach and The Marriage Mentor
Award-winning Author of HAPPY LOVE
www.TheLiftedLid.com

Foreword

Have you ever stopped to think about the health of your body at any given moment? What about the fact that the choices you are making now will affect your health in years to come?

Do you ever feel that you could be living up to a fuller potential in your body, mind and spirit?

You are meant for great things, and it is people like Francisca that can remind you of that.

Francisca walks the talk when it comes to health and wellness! Her journey with obstacles in her health presented an opportunity to choose to learn and grow, or just manage with the cards she had been dealt. She can certainly show you that, even in the darkest times of your life, there is an opportunity for growth, and commitment to being a better person in every aspect.

Francisca is constantly educating herself on not only how she may be leading a better life, but also how she can share this wealth of knowledge with you. Through her writing, studies and passionate drive, she is on a mission to help you examine your own life and reach your highest potential.

How I Conquered Breast Cancer Without Chemotherapy will offer guidance on how to engage with all parts of your life in a more mindful and holistic manner. This in turn will only create better health in the long run. And as Francisca quotes in the book: "Health is wealth!"

But more importantly, this book will offer hope to you, in case you need some inspiration to feel that better days are always ahead. If you commit to being the best version of yourself, you can truly do anything you put your mind to!

Raymond Aaron
New York Times Bestselling Author

Chapter 1

The Genesis

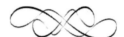

"Where there is no struggle,
there is no strength."
— **Oprah Winfrey**

1

Cancer is a disease that has affected most people's lives in one way or another. If you have not heard of someone being diagnosed with cancer, whether they are close to you or not, you have certainly been living under a rock! I jest, but it is a fact of modern life. Not only has my family been deeply impacted by this disease, I myself have as well. Unfortunately, I have lost five family members (nuclear and extended) to this disease, and I myself received my own cancer diagnosis. This disease has always been part of my life in one way or another.

After my healing journey from cancer, I felt called to share that journey with you. I now not only believe, but I **know** for a fact, that this disease does not have to be a death sentence. I want to ensure that not only my friends and family know this but that you know this as well. I want you not to feel scared of this killer lurking in the shadows. Instead, I want you to know that you have many options available to you in order to begin fighting any possibility of this disease TODAY.

I want to share with you not only my experience in confronting cancer head on, but what I learned along the way. Most people feel that this disease is something that is out of their control. But I am here to tell you, it is NOT. Cancer is not only conquerable, but it is preventable in a myriad of ways. Throughout this book I will share everything I learned on my own journey to curing my cancer without the use of traditional drugs or the usual western medicine course of action. As you read, please remember that I am not a doctor or healer. I was seeking answers and had a belief that there must be another way to manage this disease that has ravaged many lives. I am here to prove that there is another way to be cancer-free and full of vitality. I am glad you are here, and hope my story serves you and the ones you love.

The Start of My Journey

One of my mentors always stressed to me: *"If you keep doing what you have always done, you will keep getting what you have always got."* So, when it came to my cancer diagnosis, I explored the possibility of doing something different. As I mentioned before, this disease had already found its way into my life by taking the lives of those I loved. So, all I saw was a possibility of taking another road to managing this disease, as I was determined that it would not be the end of life. Furthermore, I wanted to put an end to the generational curse of losing family members from this fatal disease.

Back in October 2014, one week before travelling to Asia, I was working with a homeopathic doctor who ended up diagnosing my right breast as "not functioning well." Because I was in the process of travelling, I just dismissed the notion, as it was not a top priority at that time. I do my breast self-examinations religiously and urge everyone to do them! If you are of childbearing age, both women AND men should be doing these important monthly self-checks as mammograms are not one hundred percent accurate. Mammograms do not detect all types of cancer in the breast.

While I was living in the USA, one day I did feel a lump in my right breast. I immediately sought an opinion from my doctor who simply said that I had "dense breasts" and there was nothing to worry about. I trusted the opinion of a medical professional but of course continued the practice of doing self-examinations. After several years, having moved to Canada, I did again feel a new type of lump in my breast. However, this time it felt different. I went back to my doctor's opinion and simply chalked it up to the fact that I had "dense breasts" and did not react to it immediately. But after several months, I could feel that this lump grew in size, and that is when alarm bells went off in my mind. I knew in my gut that this was more than just a diagnosis of "dense breast" tissue.

I immediately booked an appointment with my family doctor. I shared what I had discovered and, yes, they confirmed that I had a lump in my right breast. I immediately went in for a mammogram and ultrasound to get a proper diagnosis of what was happening in my body. The doctor's assistant called me the next morning and told me the doctor wanted to see me right away. From the tone of her voice, I could tell that the news I was about to receive was not going to be positive.

Diagnosis

I will never forget August 1, 2019. This is the day I was diagnosed with breast cancer. When the doctor told me the news, you could hear a pin drop. We were both clearly upset. They recorded a detailed account of my family's history with cancer to gain a better understanding of what we were up against. I was referred to a top oncologist at one of the best cancer hospitals in Canada. We did all necessary tests and again I was given a positive breast cancer diagnosis. More specifically a Stage 2 diagnosis, which indicates that the disease was detected in its early stages. Immediately my thoughts went to Dr. Debra Williams, ND. Dr Williams is a naturopathic doctor, and medical missionary in Jamaica who also had Stage 2 breast cancer and cured it without chemotherapy. She became my inspiration! I knew there was light at the end of the tunnel.

I opted not to have a mastectomy (a surgical operation to remove a breast) and chose the second option of having the lump removed and a sentinel node biopsy, in order to determine if the cancer had spread to any other parts of my body. I was elated to learn that it had not! The next step was to begin rounds of chemotherapy, followed by radiation treatments. However, after learning the news that the lump had not spread, I boldly exercised my patient's bill of rights and opted NOT to have chemotherapy. Of course, this is an unusual move that was not taken lightly by my oncologist. "I have been an oncologist for twenty-five years and none of my patients have ever refused chemotherapy treatment," he told me, maybe in the hope that I would change my mind, or to ensure that I knew I was really going against the grain.

I did not take this choice lightly. But I was very sure. I remembered the words, *"If you keep doing what you have always done, you will keep getting what you have always got"* in this situation. I felt deep down that if I followed the conventional path it would lead to the same fate of my relatives: not surviving this disease.

I enlisted a holistic doctor to help me with this new leg of my journey, and off we went. Fast forward a year later to August 2020, when I had a follow-up breast ultrasound and mammogram with my oncologist. He examined my right breast and exclaimed, "Whatever that doctor did to you, he or she did a good job!" I could not help but smile like a Cheshire cat! It has now been over 2 years since my cancer diagnosis and I am happy to report that my breast cancer remains in remission.

Now that you have a snapshot of my whole cancer story, I am looking forward to diving into some work with you. I want to share with you everything I learned on this journey that took me from the possibility of living (or dying) with a disease to being cancer-free. Today I feel I am in the best health I have ever been, and I wish that for you and your loved ones as well. Whether you are fighting the disease now or just want to be mindful and live in a more preventable way, I want to show you that great health is obtainable no matter from where you are starting. Let us dive in!

Setting Yourself Up and Starting From Where You Are

If you are ever to face adversity, be it a battle with cancer or something else, you have to set yourself up right to really have the strength to fight. Of course, there is a physical strength component. However, most of what you need to harness is the **mental strength** to withstand this battle. It can be a long and challenging journey to regain your full health. At the end of the day, it comes down to having the proper mindset.

I want to share with you some starting points to gain perspective on what I developed and then took with me throughout my journey. The most important thing in this moment is to remember to start from where you are. Start exactly from whatever mindset and mental attitude you have and become committed to expanding that to be the best you can be.

Positive Mental Attitude

"Two men looked out from prison bars;
one saw mud, the other saw stars."
- Dale Carnegie

I feel this quote perfectly depicts how I was feeling during my cancer journey, especially when I was first diagnosed. Having cancer made me feel like I was a prisoner. A prisoner to my body and this diagnosis. Suddenly my life was identified in a different light. However, just as the prisoner who looked out of the prison cell and saw stars, I was hopeful.

Someone close to me was also going through his own cancer battle at the time. He gave me the best advice when he advised me to stay hopeful, no matter what, as it would help with my healing process. That first piece of advice was invaluable, especially knowing what I know

now. A healing process rooted in hope is essential when facing this disease. Hope is one factor of having a positive mental attitude.

Positive mental attitude (PMA) is a concept first introduced by Napoleon Hill in 1937 in the popular book, *Think and Grow Rich.* This concept has since been adopted by many who want to create change in their life. When you have the right mental attitude in any situation, it attracts positive change and results in your life. Having a developed and strong PMA is essential when managing cancer.

Studies have been done which clearly show a correlation to patients having a strong positive mental attitude and recovering from illness faster, as opposed to patients who view life with a more negative gaze. I can definitely attest to this personally. Not only did I have my own developed sense of positivity, I was also surrounded by positive support. I have warm memories of my siblings sending me flowers and cards to show their support. I appreciated these kind gestures more than they could imagine. When I saw their gifts, I was always reminded to come back to a positive place in my mind.

Starting from where you are, do you feel that you carry a positive mindset or do you tend to live in a more negative state? Wherever you are at, even if you feel you are generally a positive person, it is always a good idea to continue to cultivate a positive mental attitude within. This will enable you to continue on your journey, whether it is fighting disease or whatever else life throws at you, with great hope.

Visualizations

Visualizations are a very powerful tool that you can use for many things in your life.

You may have already heard about using visualizations in your life. During the journey of healing my cancer, I would harness the power of visualization and see myself being healed and cancer-free in my mind's eye multiple times a day. This kept me inspired and driven, and also acted as a guiding post for my body. Through visualizing that I was healthy, I gave subconscious ideas and guidance to my body. I was directing it to the state I wanted it to be in: cancer-free!

Beyond visualizing with your mind, there are other techniques, such as creating a vision or dream board. A vision board is a collection of images, words, phrases and colors, either assembled altogether onto one board or simply pinned individually onto a board. The images represent what you want to BE, DO and HAVE. You create a snapshot of your future. It is fun to have images pinned separately on a board so that you can transfer them to a "completion" board when you have achieved them. Another great visualization tool is to have your goals written on individual cards that you can read throughout the day. These cards are easily transportable and can help keep your mind focused on aligning with your goals.

As you can see, this is a powerful all-round tool to use for your life. When you are using visualization to improve your health or rid yourself of a disease as I was using it, it becomes another important piece of a larger puzzle that will help lead you to heal your body and create better health.

Affirmations

In addition to visualizations, many successful people also use affirmations as part of their daily practices that keep them in a positive mindset and set themselves up for greatness. Before my cancer diagnosis, I already had a daily practice of both visualizations and affirmations, so I felt a bit more prepared when I needed to pivot the core reason.

Affirmations are sayings or quotes that you recite to yourself every day in order to elevate your positive energy. They create an opportunity for you to connect to thoughts and feelings that make you feel good, or feeling better than you currently do.

I want to share with you some of my favorite affirmations that have really helped me. They keep me feeling positive and grounded. During my battle with cancer, I welcomed them into my life wholeheartedly:

- I praise you because I am fearfully and wonderfully made. (Psalm 139:14) NIV
- I trust you wholeheartedly and surrender my life to your guidance.
- God grant me the strength to change what I can, the courage to accept what I can't, and wisdom to know the difference. (Serenity Prayer)
- I am open to receiving. I remain patient, positive, loving and faithful.

Do you have any affirmations that inspire you? You may have one or several. They may come from different sources or people. The most important thing is that when you recite them, they make you feel alive, hopeful and ready to overcome any adversity you may be facing. Or they can simply act as a boost to your energy every day. If you currently do not have any affirmations that you practice, I encourage you to find at least one that may serve you moving forward!

Possible Causes of Cancer

The conversation around what causes cancer is extensive. As I mentioned in this book, I will be discussing lifestyle choices that I found contributed directly to me taking my health back from this horrible disease. It is incredibly eye-opening at how empowered we are when bringing ourselves to a high, positive state of health. Beyond what I will speak about are a few things worth mentioning that I want to draw attention to. You can then choose to begin your own research on these specific aspects if you wish.

Starting with examining your diet is essential, and one of the very first things that you can do immediately. Do you eat a lot of processed food or fresh whole food? I will go into detail about foods I have been eating to stay healthy as well as discuss general quantity and frequency of eating in another chapter. But let me first plant a seed in your mind with the question I asked.

A few larger, more broad topics I will not be covering in depth in this book as you can literally write full books on certain cancer-causing elements alone. I must briefly mention them, though, so that you can further investigate for yourself.

The environment you live in can directly affect your health. You may not be aware of how many pollutants are actually surrounding you at any given moment. From transportation to agriculture to everyday household activities, you are constantly exposed to chemicals that affect your health. You will never be able to avoid them all together. However, when you begin to understand how large of a scale this is, you can then take care of the things that you may actually be able to control (a lot of that is covered in this book.) When it comes down to it, pollutants are not naturally occurring aspects of your environment, so they can be detrimental to your health.

Genetics can play a part in the possibility of getting cancer at some point in your life. Take myself for example. I believe this is how I ended up with breast cancer. As I mentioned in my dedication, I have had five people in my family die because of the disease. So in hindsight it does not surprise me that I ended up with a cancer diagnosis.

In our modern world there is one thing that is very difficult to escape: stress! Stress can come in many forms from minor to major, and can be seen as a very large part of the many ways your health can malfunction. It is multifaceted and can at times be complicated. While you will most likely never be able to truly escape stress altogether, the key will be to manage it properly. Based on studies that I read about via City of Hope (www.cityofhope.org), chronic stress can provoke cancer to spread quicker (especially in breast, colorectal and ovarian cancer). Science says that when our bodies become tired and stressed out, neurotransmitters such as norepinephrine (also a stress hormone) are released into the body, which stimulates cancer cells. So imagine if you are constantly under a steady hum of stress. Chronic stress is no joke, and it is up to you to understand your stress and learn how to manage as soon as possible. Your life may depend on it!

I am so grateful you are here and wanting to learn more about my journey. It means you care about yourself and your loved ones, and believe in the possibility of not only being cancer-free, but also believe in living a healthy and energized life in general. The first part of my healing journey was to change some simple lifestyle choices that might not seem like a lot, but at the end of the day really are game changers.

Chapter 2

Necessary Lifestyle Changes

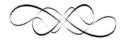

"Change will not come if we wait for some other person or some other time. We are the ones we have been waiting for. We are the change that we seek."
— **Barack Obama**

was off on my journey to heal my body and rid myself of breast cancer. I decided to work closely with a holistic health practitioner who wanted to create a focus on changing aspects of my lifestyle that could be negatively contributing to my health. We identified the elements of my life that needed major overhaul and some that just simply required a bit of tweaking. Our goal was to change habits, improve my health, and then allow myself to fight the cancer in my body. I will outline some of the first changes I easily implemented right away. When I first implemented them, I of course was doing it because of my diagnosis. But, dear reader, you do not have to wait until you are sick to take on anything I discuss in this chapter or beyond. I actually urge you to take everything in this book to heart and begin to understand that there is something to be said for preventative measures.

Personal Care Products

The first things I want to look at are the numerous everyday personal care products that are a part of your grooming and hygiene routines. I bet that many of you reading this will relate to the fact that you may be using more conventional items without even a thought as to what is actually in these products, let alone how they are affecting your body. My holistic health practitioner had me immediately replace the items listed below with naturally derived ones. It was a whole new world for me, but I eagerly embraced these changes because I wanted to be healed from my breast cancer using more unorthodox methods. I felt that my holistic doctor wanted me to be healed as much as I did. My thoughts and feelings were that of optimism, because I felt that if Dr Debra Williams, ND, could be healed from Stage 2 cancer using natural methods, I too could be healed!

Body Lotion

Applying lotion to your body after a shower can help bring much nourishment to your skin. It keeps it hydrated, soft and smooth. It is advisable that you try to use lotion that is formulated for your specific skin type; however, many lotions can be used for multiple types of skin.

Finding a new, all-natural lotion for yourself may sometimes be a complicated process. My holistic doctor suggested that I use a certain type of extra virgin oil at first. I invested in it and began trying it as part of my daily personal care routine. However, it reacted adversely with my skin. So afterwards I was recommended a lotion that was a beautiful combination of tea tree oil, rice bran oil, glycerin oil, primrose oil, jojoba oil, almond oil, castor oil, avocado oil, olive oil, coconut oil and organic shea butter. This lotion not only felt amazing, but after doing some more research on the ingredients I also learned that their benefits went beyond just moisturizing my skin. How incredible!

I have to be transparent with you and share that this lotion was more of a financial investment that I was used to making. I was used to simply going to the drug store or other beauty supply places and buying whatever I wanted, or whatever was on sale. When you choose to buy all-natural and high-quality products for your skin, the price point may go up. This is just a fact of switching from a mass manufactured lotion to a high-quality product. But I am more than happy to pay more for my health. Plus, I found my skin to be so much more nurtured and healthier looking after I switched. Truly this is the best I have ever used!

Deodorant

I use deodorant daily as most of you do as well, no doubt! It is such a regular part of our personal hygiene that you may not even think about it. Applying your deodorant is just as automatic as brushing your teeth. Another recommendation for my lifestyle that was made by the holistic health practitioner was to immediately implement was to replace my deodorant with a natural one.

Now I did not even know this existed. Were all these products not the same? Again, it came down to the ingredients and how they could be harmful to my body. The best choice for your health is to choose a deodorant that contains NO aluminum, propylene glycol or artificial fragrance. The first thing to focus on is the adverse effects of aluminum. Aluminum is found in any conventional deodorant that is labelled as an "antiperspirant." I was cautioned against using any deodorant with this ingredient as it has been linked to Alzheimer's disease, neurotoxicity (adversely affecting the central or peripheral nervous system) and breast cancer. Considering my situation, the breast cancer component piqued my interest first, and I learned that the aluminum will enter the bloodstream through the skin and over time build up on breast tissue, which can eventually cause cancer.

I was shocked that this one particular ingredient could actually cause this amount of harm in the body. When I did some more research on the other ingredients, such as propylene glycol, I learned that many have direct links to acute and chronic health issues, including cancer. Again, imagine the amazing changes that you can be creating in your body by simply replacing one product with a naturally derived one? The natural deodorant market has certainly expanded in recent years. If you have friends that use a natural deodorant, inquire as to which brands they like, or begin your journey to find which one works for you. Look for aluminum free, propylene glycol free and artificial fragrance free. Because every one of us has different body chemistry, you may have to try a few to find one that works for you. But going through this process is worth it! You are creating positive and lasting change in your health.

Toothpaste

I brush my teeth up to three times a day. An astonishing fact that I learned from my holistic doctor is that the usual toothpaste you buy from the drug or grocery store is harmful for your health! It can actually be dangerous. If you look at the fine print on toothpastes it will clearly state "DO NOT SWALLOW" and that if more is swallowed than needed for brushing, you should seek medical attention. This warning alone opened my eyes and caused a stir in me. It does not make sense that a product that I have to put in my mouth in order to use it could be dangerous in any way if swallowed.

My holistic doctor advised me to simply begin using aluminum free baking soda as a toothpaste. At first I thought she was joking but she was dead serious! Again, as with everything there was an adjustment. This may have felt like the biggest one. Not only was the texture and taste totally different than what I was used to, I also had to get the idea out of my head that "proper" toothpaste had to be foamy, taste a certain way, and be filled with all the chemicals that your conventional ones are. Being as committed as I was, I stuck with it and never looked back. I am used to it now and do not even think about just using baking soda. It is my new normal, and I know that if I can do it so can you! Why would you continue to use a product that could harm you in such a vulnerable area as your mouth? Even when it clearly says it could, right on the label?

In The Home

Moving away from personal care, let us take a look at the next set of action items that I was asked to change immediately in order to begin creating a healthier environment for my body to heal in. Outside of personal care products there are many parts of usual daily routines that you need to be mindful of changing. The conventional way may not be the healthiest way. I want to share with you a few things that you can change right now that will stop the cycle of harming your body. This is all about not bringing more "pollution" into the home, so that your body can function optimally.

Stop Using a Microwave

One of the first changes I made when it came to daily habits in the kitchen was to stop using a microwave altogether. When I learned about the harmful radiation that microwaves emit, I immediately ceased using mine in my home. And later when I moved homes, I decided not to have a microwave in my new kitchen at all. There was an adjustment at first, no doubt. The microwave was introduced in the 1950's as a high-tech addition to the kitchen, and with its evolution in design eventually became a mainstay in kitchens all over the world. People were sold on its convenience, and if you grew up with a microwave you might not be able to imagine your life without one. However, choosing not to use a microwave, or even getting rid of the one in your kitchen a together, is a definitive way of keeping harmful radiation out of your home.

When I was advised to stop using my microwave altogether it certainly took some getting used to! No more microwaved meals or reheating things with the click of a button and being able to just walk away. But as I wanted to improve my health as best I could, I started doing all the cooking and reheating of food in the oven or on the stove top. Changing this habit took a bit of forethought at first but I adapted more quickly than I expected. My friends and family now also know that when they come to visit there is no microwave. Funny how even for them it was a change but of course they know the "why" behind my decision and respect it fully.

Use Parchment Paper

Parchment paper has become a staple in my kitchen when I use the oven. This is a specific type of paper that has been created to be moisture and grease resistant as well as being able to withstand higher temperatures. It comes in sheets or a roll, and can be found in the section of your grocery store where the wax paper or plastic wrap may be. Many people know parchment as a great tool for lining and when baking cookies or something similar. However, I now use it for everything.

In my cooking habits, parchment paper took the place of using any aluminum foil. As we already examined earlier, aluminum is harmful to your body. So, I immediately switched to parchment paper and it took aluminum foil's place. I use it for cooking, baking or reheating anything in the oven. It is extremely easy to use and cleans up easily. I am amazed that it is another small change that we can all implement and one that, over time, may greatly affect our health.

Household Cleaning Products

The third household related habit I immediately changed under the advice of my holistic practitioner was to use only all-natural cleaners in my home. Conventional cleaners that you have for things like countertops to bathrooms to floors to windows all contain harsh chemicals and compounds that essentially pollute your home. When you use them, you are introducing these chemicals into your immediate environment and exposing yourself to them. When making the switch, look for all-purpose cleaners made from plant-based ingredients which are biodegradable.

There is an extensive market for natural household cleaners. You can replace every cleaning solution you have with one that is naturally derived. However, with some research I also discovered many homemade cleaning solutions that are made with ingredients you may already have in your home. In fact, The Organic Consumers Association lists baking soda, borax, lemon juice, soap, vinegar and water as "safe" cleaners. For example, I now use white vinegar as part of many of the cleaning products that I make myself. Not only is it inexpensive, but it has many uses beyond being used in your cooking. Vinegar is non-toxic and eco-friendly, making it the ultimate multipurpose cleaning solution. In most cases, you only need to mix vinegar with water to create your own all-purpose cleaner. Some common uses of vinegar are: appliances, bath tubs, countertops, dishwashers, faucets, floors, glass, laundry, showers, sinks and toilets. {source: Debra Rose Wilson, PhD, RN. Vinegar: The Multi-purpose, Chemical-free Household Cleaner You Should Know About.}

Like all changes we have been talking about, it may take some time to adapt to this new habit. But always remember the reason you are doing it -- for the health of you and your loved ones. Your cleaning products do NOT have to be full of dangerous and harsh chemicals in order to be effective.

As you continue to do your own research, I know you will be as surprised as I was at how many uses there are for things such as different vinegars. Many ingredients are so powerful and multifaceted that you will be able to help yourself in countless ways as you start on your journey to rid your home of toxic chemicals. Beyond saving your health and even some money, I bet you end up wondering why you had not been incorporating these new ways of being a long time ago. Well, I congratulate you for being here now, and making the changes now. It is never too late to start a new chapter and commit to the betterment of your health!

I have covered some basics with you of switching personal care and household products that are full of chemicals and toxins, to ones that are all-natural and safe for your health. Let us now focus on your diet. I want to look at what you are eating, how much and when. There are also many supplements that you can be taking in order to achieve optimal health. Again, this is all based on the changes that I implemented in my life that helped me cure my breast cancer, and now feel the best I have in years! Let us first look at food, and what we can be eating to enhance our nutrition. I cannot stress how important this is.

Chapter 3

Holistic Nutrition

"The first wealth is health."
— Ralph Waldo Emerson

3

You may be familiar with the popular saying: "**You are what you eat.**" When it comes to nutrition this can very much be taken to heart. Our bodies will absorb the properties of the foods and drinks we ingest. When it comes down to it, it is quite simple: if you want to be healthy, you must eat healthy foods. If you want to be unhealthy, then keep reaching for foods that are highly processed or unbalanced. Take a moment now and reflect on what you choose to eat. You may never have really thought about it before, and in that case, I am glad you are here! Maybe you try to avoid certain things but do not pay attention to the full picture of everything you eat in a day. When it comes to what you choose to eat, you have to stop looking at food just as something to quell your hunger. Your food is fuel! You must change your perspective from food being something you just eat, to being the nutrients and nutrition you require in order to have great health. In the bigger picture, eliminating many of the "comfort foods" in your diet is a small price to pay in order to stop the growth and spread of cancer.

When I was diagnosed with breast cancer, I knew that part of the puzzle to my recovery would be changing my diet. As with everything else I was changing in my life, it was evident that every aspect of my life including my dietary choices were affecting my health (and obviously not for the better). I wanted to learn what to eat in order to optimally function and to allow my body to heal itself. If you are what you eat, I wanted to be healthy!

I sought the services of a dietician. Together we examined what my usual eating habits had been like, and then examined my goals. Because I was looking for foods to fight and prevent cancer, they recommended a very specific food plan for me: G.B.O.M.B.S, which stands for Greens, Beans, Onions, Mushrooms, Berries, Seeds. This type of eating plan consists of whole foods, free of anything processed, and each food has specific properties that would help me in my fight against cancer. At the end of the day though, the nutrition that this specific diet holds is excellent for anyone! In addition to eating these foods I was advised to cut out dairy, meat, sugar and wheat (which I definitely found hard at first)!

I have many healthcare providers in my family, so I had been mindful of healthy eating all my life, and up until this point it had served me well. I felt healthy and have always looked younger than my actual age. So much so that I have even been courted by men who were too young for me, because they thought I was about 15 years younger than I actually was! But approaching a diet from this point of view was still a shift. I was now eating to serve my health, not just maintain it. I was looking to create change in my body and was going to use these potent foods as medicine in a way, not just something good to eat.

I will share with you the specific benefits of each food group individually, and provide a sample list of foods. This will give you some insight into understanding how each group individually can help your body to be nourished and working optimally to fight and prevent cancer.

Greens

Green vegetables are the first item on the list of this diet of holistic nutrition. My late mother trained as a registered nurse. Because of this, as far back as I can remember when we were toddlers, our parents instilled in us the importance of healthy eating. I am lucky as I have always loved vegetables so I had no problem incorporating even more into my diet.

What makes green vegetables so good for you is the chlorophyll. Chlorophyll is a green pigment that helps vegetables produce and absorb more nutrients when going through photosynthesis. It is considered a natural source of antioxidants. Antioxidants in your diet are necessary in preventing and fighting cancer as they protect your cells from free radicals (which are cancer causing agents). Green vegetables also contain high amounts of magnesium and iron. Other great health benefits besides preventing cancer include:

- Controlling blood pressure
- Strengthening your bones
- Preventing heart disease
- Improving your vision
- Boosting your immune system
- Rehydrating the body
- Aiding in weight loss
- Treating constipation
- Reducing the risk of diabetes

(Source: 10 Health Benefits of Green Vegetables by Dr. Michelle Heben)

Sample list of green vegetables:

- Artichoke
- Arugula
- Asparagus
- Bell Pepper
- Bitter Gourd
- Broccoli
- Brussels Sprouts
- Calabash

- Celery
- Chayote
- Coriander
- Cucumber
- Edamame
- Grape Leaves
- Green Beans
- Green Chili Pepper
- Green Pumpkin
- Kale
- Kohlrabi
- Leeks
- Lettuce
- Microgreens
- Okra
- Peas
- Perilla
- Ridge Gourd
- Spinach
- Watercress
- Zucchini

Beans

I have always understood that beans are very healthy, but I used to avoid eating them often because I would get bloated. When I lived in the United States, a former co-worker shared with me a secret from his grandmother to help prevent bloating and passing wind after eating beans. He instructed me to cook beans with one big unpeeled Irish potato. Well, I tried it and bingo! It worked like magic. Years later, I also learned online that putting a quarter teaspoon of baking soda to one pound of beans will help to prevent any gaseous side effects from eating beans. This also worked like a charm. If you usually experience these sort of side effects from eating beans try either of these methods and I am sure they will work for you as well!

Also known as legumes or peas, beans are seeds from the Fabaceae family. They are high in fiber, iron and numerous vitamins. Beans are also a great plant-based protein, which is nice when trying to cut down or cut out animal product consumption. Besides being a great food that contributes to cancer prevention, they also have many health benefits that include:

- Contains folate (a type of B vitamin)
- Contains antioxidants
- Improving heart health
- Managing diabetes & glucose metabolism
- Preventing fatty liver
- Helping to control your appetite
- Improving gut health

(Source: Medical News Today)

Sample list of beans:

- Adzuki Beans
- Anasazi Beans
- Black Beans
- Black-eyed Peas
- Cannellini Beans
- Chickpeas
- Cranberry Beans
- Fava Beans
- Flageolet Beans
- Great Northern Beans
- Kidney Beans
- Lentils

- Lima Beans
- Mung Beans
- Navy Beans
- Peas
- Pinto Beans
- Red Beans
- Soybeans

Onions

One day when I was working as a hostess in the faculty club while pursuing my postgraduate studies in the United States, my friends and I were chatting about different food items. One of them brought up the old adage of "An apple a day keeps the doctor away." Another co-worker shared that her grandmother used to eat a raw onion daily and she was never sick. Someone then exclaimed: "An onion a day keeps *everyone* away!" Everyone laughed as onions definitely have and probably always will have a reputation for their pungent aroma and taste.

When it came to increasing my onion intake, I did not see it as a challenge at all. I really do not mind the taste of onions, and I was committed to getting better.

Onions are a unique food as they are cultivated and consumed across the globe. They are generally a temperate crop; however, they can be grown in all sorts of conditions. Usually served cooked, they can also be eaten raw, or served in pickles or chutneys. Onions are a key food when preventing or fighting cancer. A study done by the University of Guelph showed that red onions were the most effective when it came to destroying breast and colon cancer cells. This is because of the high levels of quercetin and anthocyanin, two compounds that directly contribute to this effect. Onions on a whole activate the pathways that provoke the cancer cells to kill themselves, and create an unfavourable environment for cancer to grow. As the cancer cells have difficulty communicating, this inhibits their growth. Some other notable benefits of eating onions are:

- Preventing inflammation and other allergies
- Promoting healthy digestion
- Promoting respiratory health
- Reducing oxidative stress in the body
- Lowering blood sugar levels
- Enhancing brain health
- Fights cancer… and many more!

(Source: 31 Surprising Benefits of Onions for Skin, Hair and Health by Ravi Teja Tadimalla)

Sample list of onions:

- Bermuda Onions
- Boiling Onions
- Chives
- Cipollini Onions
- Cocktail Onions
- Creole Onions
- Egyptian Onions
- Green Onions
- Leeks
- Maui Onions
- Mayan Sweet Onions
- Owa Onions
- Pearl Onions
- Pickling Onions
- Red Onions
- Red Wing Onions
- Shallots
- Spanish Onions
- Texas "Supa Sweet" Onions

- Torpedo Onions
- Tropea Lunga Onions
- Vidalia Onions
- Walla Walla Sweet Onions
- Welsh Onions
- White Onions
- Yellow Onions

Mushrooms

I used to eat mushrooms sparingly because I found them to be quite tasteless, especially when eaten raw in salads. But I was committed to adding as many of them as I could into my diet. I still feel they do not have much taste on their own unless they are seasoned very well. I have also learned how to incorporate them into great recipes that are now part of my regular weekly meals.

Mushroom (or toadstools) are the fleshy body of a fungus, typically produced above ground, on soil, or on their food source. They can be found growing out in the wild, and are also cultivated and farmed. Mushrooms have been used as a source of holistic nutrition all over the world for centuries, due to their unique properties. Mushrooms contain immune supporting nutrients and vitamins that can help with protecting against various types of cancer and maintaining good heart health. Many of the benefits of this underrated food group may surprise you:

- Good source of selenium (a powerful antioxidant)
- Can help improve cholesterol
- Promotes improved gut health
- Boosts immunity
- Contain anti-inflammatory properties
- Good source of fiber
- Rich source of B vitamins

- Contain anti-cancer properties... and more!

(Source: 10 Surprising Health Benefits of Eating Mushrooms - Shalini Adams, Daily Health Body)

Sample list of mushrooms:

- Beef Steak Mushrooms
- Button Mushrooms
- Calocybe Gambosa Mushrooms
- Cauliflower Mushrooms
- Chanterelle Mushrooms
- Clamshell Mushrooms
- Cremini Mushrooms
- Enoki Mushrooms
- Hedgehog Mushrooms
- Jack-o-lantern Mushrooms
- King Oyster Mushrooms
- Lobster Mushrooms
- Maitake Mushrooms
- Meadow Mushrooms
- Milk Mushrooms
- Morel Mushrooms
- Pine Mushrooms
- Porcini Mushrooms
- Portobello Mushrooms
- Russula Mushrooms
- Shiitake Mushrooms
- St. George's Mushrooms
- White Mushrooms
- Wood Blewit Mushrooms

Berries

Eating lots of different fruits has been a cornerstone of my diet for as long as I can remember. In my teen years we had several fruit trees on the property where we lived. We enjoyed mangoes, guavas, pineapples and others! My mother used to always bring extra fruits to the hospital where she worked to give to patients to help supplement their diets. She would also encourage us to take fruits to school to share with friends. I am known to always have some fresh fruit in my bag, and actually prefer eating fruit as opposed to just reaching for a painkiller at the onset of a headache. I find this simple remedy very effective for me. For this diet I was asked to specifically focus on eating berries.

Berries are small, round, juicy, pulpy, edible fruits. Depending on the type of berry, they may be found in the wild as well as cultivated and farmed. Because of their deep and rich color, berries are known to be packed with antioxidants, which as mentioned before are incredible cancer fighting agents. Cranberries specifically have compounds which are known to be potent cancer preventers. Berries are also a good source of fiber and contain incredible amounts of folate (B vitamins). Other amazing benefits of berries include:

- Help manage and prevent diabetes
- Can help prevent mental decline
- All berries can help prevent heart disease
- May help prevent Alzheimer's disease
- Cranberries can prevent cancer... and more!

(Source: 15 Amazing Health Benefits of Berries by Joseph Hindy)

Sample list of berries:

- Acai Berries
- Black Currants

- Black Raspberries
- Blackberries
- Blueberries
- Boysenberries
- Buffalo Berries
- Cape Gooseberries
- Chokeberries
- Cloudberries
- Cranberries
- Elderberries
- Goji Berries
- Golden Raspberries
- Gooseberries
- Huckleberries
- Lingonberries
- Mulberries
- Muscadine Berries
- Olalla Berries
- Pine Berries
- Red Currants
- Red Raspberries
- Salmon Berries
- Strawberries
- White Raspberries

Seeds

Seeds and nuts belong to the same family. I feel grateful as I have not encountered any digestive problems eating either. Seeds are an incredible food. Essentially, they are embryonic plants that are enclosed in protective coverings. Seeds are generally high in antioxidants and healthier fats that help in nourishing the brain and body, which is why they can be fantastic at preventing cancer. They are a beautiful whole food and an easy addition to any diet.

Here are also some other benefits of seeds:

- A good source of dietary fiber (which is essential for healthy digestion)
- Reduces the levels of inflammation in the body (which starves off aging and reduces the risk of heart disease)
- If consumed regularly, seeds can help prevent weight loss over time

(Source: The Health Benefits of Seeds-Why You Need to Eat Them by Nishita Kaushik)

Sample list of seeds:

- African eggplant Seeds
- Anise Seeds
- Ataiko Seeds
- Black Seeds
- Caraway Seeds
- Chia Seeds
- Coriander Seeds
- Cucumber Seeds
- Egusi Seeds
- Fennel Seeds
- Fenugreek Seeds
- Flax Seeds
- Hemp Seeds
- Iregege Seeds
- Melon Seeds
- Muskmelon Seeds
- Ogbonna Seeds
- Pine Nuts
- Pomegranate Seeds
- Poppy Seeds
- Pumpkin Seeds
- Quinoa Seeds

- Sesame Seeds
- Sunflower Seeds
- Uziza Seeds
- Watermelon Seeds
- Wild Seeds
- Yellow Mustard Seeds

Even after my breast cancer was eradicated, I kept following the G.B.O.M.B.S. diet. Not only because I am committed to preventing any future cancers developing, but it also makes me feel full of energy. It helps my body feel great, and I also noticed it helps keep my mind clear as well. I know that for most of you, trading in your usual foods for a diet of this nature may be a huge change. Remember that you do not have to do it all at once. You can work on the diet slowly but surely introducing more of the specified foods and then committing to making the full overhaul.

It is just a fact of life that most of the time we have to use supplements in our diets in order to actually intake a full spectrum of vitamins and minerals. Sometimes we may also need to take certain herbs for their specific health benefits. I want to share with you the supplementation regimen that I was advised to follow for beating my breast cancer. It is eye opening to understand how specific supplements really can make a huge difference in your overall health.

Chapter 4

Supplements

"I believe that you can, by taking some simple and inexpensive measures, lead a longer life and extend your years of well-being. My most important recommendation is that you take vitamins every day in optimum amounts to supplement the vitamins that you receive in your food."
— Linus Pauling

F ood supplements are concentrated sources of nutrients (vitamins and minerals) or other herbs that have specific physiological and psychological effects on the body. Each supplement has a recommended dose that it is administered in, and should be followed carefully as there can be such a thing as "too much of a good thing." All supplements can be found over the counter at your local pharmacy or health food store. They are not regulated by the US Food and Drug Administration, so it is imperative that you buy your supplements from trusted and reputable brands.

Taking your vitamins can go so far beyond just popping a multi-vitamin and being done for the day. It can be seen as another way to support your body and all its systems, so that you can lead an optimally healthy life. Based on the state of my failing health when I began fighting my cancer, of course I was up for adding any and all supplements to my diet. I actually almost expected to, as I already understood how powerful they could be. My holistic practitioner strongly advised me to follow a list of daily supplements in order to strengthen my immune system. Again, these recommended supplements were specific to what I was trying to accomplish health-wise.

You may be wondering why, if I was following a strict G.B.O.M.B.S. diet, I would need additional supplements. Supplements can make up for the fact that some nutrients are lost when you cook your food. Also, it is very helpful if you cannot eat all your food from organic sources as some fruits and vegetables may be sprayed with preservatives for transportation to the grocery store. I always try to buy all my fresh produce from the farmers market in the summer, so I am taking the freshest and most available source of nutrients that I can. Here are some other very important reasons why some people may take supplements:

- Filling in any nutritional gaps (based on food availability or poor eating habits)
- Nutrient absorption declines with age
- Regular exercise can increase nutrient needs
- Depletion of nutrients in the soil
- Preventative measures to more expensive health issues down the road

(Source: Whole Health since 1997, December 16, 2020)

You are more than welcome to try any and all supplements. Most can be safe as long as you follow the directions listed on the label. However, if you are new to using supplements, I recommend that you consult with a natural health practitioner before starting.

Vitamin B

Taking a Vitamin B complex was the first on the list of supplements to incorporate into my daily routine. A Vitamin B complex is a specific mixture of B vitamins that is dosed specifically to each one, but altogether in one capsule. You see, each B vitamin has different properties that will affect the body differently. Perhaps you did not know that there are more than one B vitamin? Yes, there are! A snapshot of a B vitamin complex will include:

- B-1 (thiamine)
- B-2 (riboflavin)
- B-3 (niacin)
- B-5 (pantothenic acid)

- B-6 (pyridoxine)
- B-7 (biotin)
- B-9 (folic acid)
- B-12 (cobalamin)

As I mentioned, each B vitamin can play a very specific role in the body. For my purposes, I was taking it for my cell health and immune system. Other ways that B vitamin complex may affect your overall health are:

- Improving energy levels
- Stimulating growth of red blood cells
- Encouraging healthy brain function
- Assisting your cardiovascular health
- and more!

(Source: Health Line)

Vitamin C

Vitamin C is also referred to as ascorbic acid and ascorbate. It is abundant in many foods, but also offered as a dietary supplement. Vitamin C is an essential nutrient when it comes to repairing tissues in your body, and is required for the functioning of several enzymes. It is also known as one of the essential nutrients for your immune system health.

Other benefits of Vitamin C include:

- Improving mood and mental health
- Acting as an antioxidant, fights oxidative damage.
- Supporting and regenerating Vitamin E
- Increasing calcium absorption (in turn assisting with bone health)
- Enhancing the absorption of nonheme iron

- It may help to reduce the risk of cardiovascular disease

(Source: Nutrition advance, 2021)

Vitamin D3 +K2 + A

You may have heard of the benefits of Vitamin D3, especially if you live in the northern hemisphere. D3 is constantly spoken about because of its reputation for being the "sun vitamin." Essentially the only natural source of Vitamin D3 is the actual sun being absorbed by your skin, otherwise you must take a supplement! Vitamin D3 is key to many body functions such as building your immune system. However, it is now known that when you take D3, it is optimal to take it with a K2. The reason behind this is that both need to be combined in order for the D3 to be readily absorbed by your body.

When referring specifically to breast cancer, a study presented in the "American Journal of Epidemiology" (by Dr. Eric Horlick) found that when someone was exposed to more sun and had adequate vitamin D production in their young adult years, their risk for breast cancer later in adult life significantly decreased. Further research suggested that sufficient levels of Vitamin D may also reduce the risk of colorectal, prostate and pancreatic cancer, to name a few. In one study of 34,000 adults, those with high levels of Vitamin D had a 20 percent lower chance of developing all types of cancer. How incredible!

Some other benefits of Vitamin D include:

- Healthier pregnancies for moms and babies
- Wards off autoimmune disease
- Helps prevent colds and the flu
- Improves all aspects of heart health
- Boosts your mood

- Eases IBS (irritable bowel syndrome); abdominal pain, bloating, diarrhea, and constipation
- Helps protect against autism
- Increases general life expectancy
- and more!

(Source: Denise Mann- Best Health)

Vitamin E

Taking Vitamin E daily is another way to supplement your diet to include more cancer fighting power. Vitamin E is a powerful antioxidant, which as I mentioned before is a key factor in fighting free radicals in the body. Antioxidant properties protect your cells and DNA from damage that free radicals or cancer cells can cause. Vitamin E is important when it comes to supporting your vision, reproductive health and the overall health of your blood, brain and skin.

Some other benefits may include:

- Fades scars and stretch marks
- Fights wrinkles
- Protects you from sun damage
- Reduces the risk of heart disease
- Fights osteoarthritis inflammation
- Boosts your immune system
- and more!

(Source: Dr. Michelle Heben, drhealthbenefit.com)

Moringa Oleifera Capsules

Moringa Oleifera is most commonly known as Moringa. It is a plant that is native to northern India. You may have also heard it referred to as drumstick tree, horseradish tree or even ben oil tree. It comes available as a powder that you can have as a tea or in your smoothies, or as capsules. Moringa was recommended to be part of my diet for its anti-cancer effects. This is because it is packed with antioxidants which as we now know boost the immune system and protect cells from free radical damage.

Other benefits of using Moringa include:

- A potent source of vitamin C (about 7 times the amount of vitamin C you would get from eating an orange!)
- Provides 3 times the amount of iron than in a cup of spinach
- Provides 4 times the amount of vitamin A than from one carrot
- Includes potassium, calcium, and protein!
- Includes amino acids that support the immune system

(Source: Ken Wiginton medically reviewed by Melinda Ratini, DO, MS)

Red Reishi Micronized Mushroom Capsules

Remember in the last chapter when I mentioned how it was recommended to begin eating mushrooms as one of the main food groups of my new diet? Well, here we are and one of my supplements that was recommended to me is also a mushroom! My holistic practitioner never ceases to amaze me with her different protocols. I began taking Red Reishi mushrooms that had been dried and dosed specifically into capsules.

Many people regularly consume this mushroom for its potential cancer fighting properties. A study that included 4000 breast cancer survivors found that 59% regularly consumed Reishi mushrooms. Other benefits of this incredible food include:

- Boosting the immune system
- Fighting fatigue and depression
- Improving heart health
- Controlling blood sugar
- Having high antioxidant status

(Source: Healthline.com)

As you can see, the importance of supplementing your diet in different ways can be highly beneficial, especially when managing specific health issues such as fighting or preventing cancer. Engaging with a holistic practitioner and creating your own supplementation regimen may be the ticket to feeling in better health, now and in the future.

I have shared the first two steps I took when overhauling my diet. I remember when I took on the full food and supplementation plan as directed, and I felt great. I remember feeling nourished and inspired as I knew I was adding another layer of care to my day-to-day fight against my breast cancer. The third part of my diet overhaul was now ready to be introduced. I was not familiar with intermittent fasting before my holistic practitioner brought it to my attention to consider. Now I cannot imagine **not** following these guidelines to eating! Keep an open mind and let us dive into the next part of our journey.

Chapter 5

Intermittent Fasting

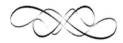

"Fasting or intermittent fasting gives us an opportunity to really get all the best cells all the time and that's what we all want."
— Dr. Steven Gundry

5

I was so excited at this point on my cancer fighting journey. At this point my life was beginning to look drastically different in terms of the choices I was making for my environment and my diet. I had one more shift to make though, when it came to my diet, and it was not about *what* I was eating, it had to do with *when* I was choosing to eat. My holistic practitioner encouraged me to try intermittent fasting in my new lifestyle. I was hesitant. I had heard of this practice, but anything to do with fasting sounded like a big undertaking. The only fasting I was familiar with was really in a more religious context and not part of a day-to-day lifestyle. But as with everything else my holistic practitioner was suggesting, I was more than willing to take on any and all changes that would assist in helping me fight my breast cancer.

I had tried fasting before, so the idea of it was not one hundred percent new to me. Of course, when I first tried fasting, it was a challenge. But eventually you do get used to it! As part of our practices at church, we would regularly fast as a congregation. Due to some pre-existing medical conditions I was managing, I was allowed to eat fruits which took "the edge" off, so to speak. I also had to be mindful as I had been managing anemia as well during some times of fasting. That was all under control before I started intermittent fasting as part of my regime to beat breast cancer. However, as we sometimes do not know one hundred percent what is going on in our bodies, it is always best to check in with your doctor or other health practitioner in order to ensure you will be set up for success.

What is Fasting?

Fasting is going without any food or drink for a specific amount of time. Fasting has commonly been known as part of religious practices or also engaged in for personal reasons. During a fast absolutely no food is taken, and usually no beverages either (and that may also include water).

Fasting is certainly not for everyone. For example, pregnant women and those with certain pre-existing medical conditions are advised not to fast. **If you are considering undertaking any sort of fasting protocol, please seek medical advice first.**

Different Types of Fasting

There are many types of fasting that all serve different purposes. I want to highlight a few so that you may then be able to distinguish them a bit better. Not only for yourself, but also to have better understanding and be supportive of anyone you may encounter who is fasting.

Absolute fast: Another name for this is "dry fasting." This fasting does not allow any water intake, along with the usual abstaining from all food and other drink.

Partial fast: This can refer to omitting one meal a day. Or it can look like only eating certain fruits and vegetables for several days at a time.

Rotational fast: Certain foods are avoided periodically. For example, grains are not eaten for several days then included in the diet for several days.

Liquid fast: Abstaining from solid food but allowing for all fluids (juices, milks, tea, water).

People engage in fasting for many different reasons. Fasts are connected to religious holidays for many different religions. They may symbolize acknowledging a particular story the holiday is centered around, or serve as a way to connect to the Divine or God. Fasting is greatly associated with a time for deep inner contemplation, and to serve as a way of better understanding oneself.

For my particular goals my holistic practitioner helped teach me about intermittent fasting and how it can be a part of my healing journey.

Why Intermittent Fasting?

You may have heard of intermittent fasting already, as it has gained popularity in recent years. As mentioned, the core idea is that you restrict all eating and drinking to only a particular time period of your day. This helps you derive some of the benefits of fasting, without having to go without food for an extended period of time. There are many forms that you can choose (in terms of the time intervals); however, "16/8" is the most popular. 16/8 is used to indicate that you fast for 16 hours and then are permitted to eat within the 8-hour window of time according to people's schedules. Many choose to eat between the hours of 12 noon and 8pm.

Benefits of Intermittent Fasting

The 16/8 intermittent fasting model is a popular diet as it is easy to follow, flexible and feels sustainable long term. Depending on what is going on in your schedule perhaps you switch your hours to a little earlier or a little later. What really counts is sticking to 16 hours of fasting during a 24-hour cycle. In terms of affecting your health, 16/8 intermittent fasting has been associated with many health benefits that include:

Increased weight loss: Because of the shorter window for eating, you will naturally cut calories as you are simply eating less. Studies have also shown that fasting for part of the day may increase metabolism and therefore help with weight loss.

Improved blood sugar control: Studies have found when regularly practicing intermittent fasting, fasting insulin levels have been reduced up to 31% and lower your blood sugar by 3-6% (all in all your overall risk of diabetes).

Longer and all-round healthier life: A recent study by Harvard researchers showed that fasting altered the mitochondrial activity in our cells. (Mitochondria are responsible for converting food into energy that the cell can use.) This may increase lifespan, slow the rate of aging and improve overall health.

(Source: Fasting: The Forgotten Cure by Josephine Marcellin)

Different Types of Intermittent Fasting

It is important to acknowledge that within the realm of intermittent fasting there are many routes you can take. I will outline them for you, but keep in mind that for my purposes of wanting to be cancer-free and prevent future cancer, I was recommended to specifically follow the 16/8 method. However, I want to provide you with as much information that I can so that you may continue to do your own investigations as to what may be right for you, depending on your health.

16/8 Method: This indicates the pattern for restricting all food intake to only an 8-hour window of 24 hrs. Beyond that you are allowed water, black coffee or tea, and any other zero calories beverages.

5/2 Diet: In this diet plan you eat normally for 5 days of your week and during the other 2 days you restrict your calories. It is recommended

500 calories for women and 600 calories for men on the 2 "fasting" days.

"Eat. Stop. Eat." Method: This involves a full fast for 24 hours once or twice a week. An example of what this may look like is to stop eating after dinner at 7pm, then to not eat until 7pm the following day. Whatever schedule works for you.

Alternate Day Fasting: This is committing to fasting every other day either by fully not eating or only eating a few hundred calories to sustain you.

Warrior Diet: This diet looks like eating a minimal amount of whole fruits and vegetables during the day then eating one large balanced meal at night. So essentially you are in a semi fast most of the day then break it at night with dinner.

(Source: Healthline.com/nutrition/6-ways-to-do-intermittent fasting)

My Personal Journey with Intermittent Fasting

As I mentioned earlier, I already had a history with fasting through my church at the time. So, engaging in intermittent fasting came a lot easier than I had expected. I still practice my 16/8 intermittent fasting, but only Monday through Friday. Now that it is just part of my maintenance plan, I allow no time restrictions on my eating during the weekend, and find that makes it a lot easier when socializing with friends or business partners.

During my journey with intermittent fasting, I noticed many positive changes with my body:

- I lost 10 pounds without focusing on that. The weight just came off.
- My body became more agile and flexible.
- I no longer experience pain in my joints.

- I no longer experience bloating as I had prior to practicing intermittent fasting.
- I am able to ingest more liquids, so staying hydrated no longer feels like a challenge.
- I have more energy! So much in fact that I am able to go for walk 30 minutes every morning AND then do another 30 minutes of aerobic exercise when I get home.
- I look and feel younger!

During a zoom conference I was tuning into, a celebrity athlete stated: "Many of you fall ill because you eat too frequently." This really piqued my interest as that sounded like a version of fasting to me. When I mentioned this statement to my holistic practitioner, she added: "And people also fall ill because they eat too much food." Dr. Miriam Merad, lead author of a new fasting study, said two meals a day may be ideal for human health. *(Source: Hilary Brueck.)* Reflecting on my own research and personal experience it is very clear to me that intermittent fasting (and other forms of fasting) have a specific and important role to play in our overall health.

In the last three chapters we have discussed everything to do with food: what to eat, when to eat, and how to supplement your diet. I hope you feel like you have a solid jumping off point to explore these aspects of healing for yourself.

As motivational speaker Zig Ziglar said, "If you help enough people get what they want, you will get what you want." I am looking forward to now jumping into talking about involving yourself in the community as a way to also heal and prevent disease.

Chapter 6

Plant Good Seeds

"We make a living by what we get,
but we make a life by what we give."
— Winston Churchill

6

P art of my life that I wanted to focus on while I was in my healing journey was giving back: not only to my community but to the world as a whole. When you give to others you raise the good energy in your life. Giving back and contributing to the world is acknowledging that you are part of a bigger picture. Your life does not just include your work, family and friends. We are all part of a bigger community, be it locally or globally.

When I began my healing journey, this became very apparent to me. Even though I was going through a challenging time, I could still take time to give back. Taking focus away from my own challenges for a while and helping lift someone else up was a necessary component of my healing. Sometimes these were actions I was already engaged in. Sometimes I found new ways to get involved. Either way it did not matter, it remains an important part of my weekly schedule.

I will share with you some ways that I give back or "plant good seeds." This is all in hope that you are then able to examine your own life and ways that you may give back if you are not already, or continue to be inspired to contribute to the community around you. Giving back fills your life on a whole with greater meaning and purpose... No wonder it was such an important part of my healing journey and continues to be a focus of mine. There are many distinct ways to contribute. Let us start with one of the most popular and easiest ways to give back, by offering your time.

Volunteering

Volunteering your time, energy and skills to a cause is such an incredible way to engage with your life. Through volunteering you directly give back to the community. At the same time, you will most certainly meet many kinds of people with different skills and talents. Taking the time to volunteer can prove to be such an effective way of expanding yourself as a person.

Volunteering usually involves putting yourself in new situations. With that comes the possibility of not only gaining new skills, but also improving your self-esteem. Taking time out of your own life to benefit the lives of others makes you feel humble and full of gratitude. Volunteering has been found to actually increase your life expectancy! *(source:breakingnewsenglish.com).* I feel the reasoning behind this is clear. When you feel useful and part of something bigger than yourself, your energy shifts to vibrate higher. It is not a coincidence that your health would be bolstered.

Also, people who give, attract good things into their lives! Maybe you have experienced this yourself. Or perhaps you know someone who always seems to attract great things into their lives, be it material or otherwise. It is simply how the world works. If you give good things, good things will come back to you.

You can seek out volunteer opportunities or you may even create your own. Get creative and always contribute in a way that feels aligned with you. To lend some inspiration, let me share with you my experience of how I came to join a team of people who focus on feeding impoverished members of my community.

My Experience of Giving Back

When I bought my new condo in October 2020, my real estate agent suggested that before I moved into the space, I ask a pastor to come by and bless this new home for me. I loved this idea! I put the word out, and a friend introduced me to a pastor who blesses homes as part of his job. The pastor arrived with his wife and the friend we had in common. After an hour of blessing my condo, reciting scriptures, reading from the Bible, taking in a mini sermon from the pastor, as well as blessing my condo with extra virgin oil and water, his wife asked me if I would like to accompany them to feed the homeless. They set up a table once a week in one of the slums in downtown Toronto where they offered a hot meal to anyone who needed one. I wholeheartedly agreed! I could not help but reflect on images of former President Barack Obama, First Lady Michelle Obama and their family helping serve at a soup kitchen on Thanksgiving Day... I felt aligned with giving back in this manner.

Spearheaded by the pastor, every Sunday we set up a table on the sidewalk and devote time to offer a nutritious, balanced meal as well as water and juice. We also offer face masks and hand sanitizers to take for personal use. One week, we noticed another group of people in the area of our table distributing sandwiches. It was incredible that another group was also organizing and giving back to those in need in our community.

It is too easy to take life for granted! After donating my time to feeding those in my community who have less than me, I am eternally grateful to The Almighty for the fact that I have food, shelter and clothing. I no longer take anything for granted, and feel blessed for all I have and all that is coming my way. I love donating my time to this cause.

Donating to Charitable Causes

There are millions of charities set up all over the world, with the goal to raise money for those in need. A charity may be large and target a larger problem or population of people. However, sometimes they are very small and specialized. There are a variety of benefits of donating to a charity, from the general to personal:

- Inspire and create civic engagement (which is so important to build health communities)
- Elevate your community standing
- Reduce your rates of stress and feel more satisfied with your life in general
- Feel more joy!
- Activate the reward center in your brain

(Source: Mary McCoy, licensed Social Worker)

I decided that I wanted to begin making a regular donation to a charity that I felt aligned with. I did some research and at the end of the day I decided to commit to donating to The Mary Kay Ash Charitable Foundation every month. The Mary Kay Ash Charitable Foundation helps carry on Mary Kay's legacy with its unified mission to support women living with cancer and to put an end to domestic violence. *(Source: About Mary Kay-Our History).* I was aware of the charity as I am a former independent Mary Kay Beauty Consultant. However, because I am an accredited community French interpreter and now a breast cancer survivor, this charity now aligns with my own goals and vision.

The Mary Kay Ash Charitable Foundation takes half their donations and provides funding to support research specifically targeted at eliminating cancers that directly affect women. Now as a breast cancer survivor, I want to be able to give back to the possibility of helping other women who do not have to go through this experience in the future.

The other half of their charitable model is in effort to end the epidemic of domestic violence against women through providing grants that assist community outreach programs as well as women's shelters. As an accredited community French interpreter, I work in many different settings which include social services. I have been called to provide interpretation in different situations at several women's shelters, the Children's Aid Society, police stations, detention centers, hospitals and other vulnerable places. I have heard firsthand the horrific stories of domestic violence and abuse that women have had to endure. I want to contribute to help end this cycle of violence against women.

As you can see, I found a charity that clearly aligns with my life and values. If you do not already have a charity that you know of that you already support or would like to, start doing some research. I am sure that there are some causes that you either personally align with, or that speak directly to your values. Find a charity that you love and could not imagine NOT giving your money to. Remember, for many charities every single dollar counts, so even if your donation is quite humble it is worth a lot. Do what you can with what you have. It is all part of planting good seeds.

Supporting Each Other

We have examined ways you can give back to the outer circles in your life. What about giving back to your more inner and personal circles? What about giving back to people who may be part of your life already, but do not necessarily need financial assistance? Perhaps there are opportunities in your life where you can give back through your time, presence and ideas. This can look like being part of a community group or perhaps even through a more professional development lens. I am lucky as I have several ways in my life that I am able to contribute to different circles or people's lives using not only my time, but also through utilizing skills I have developed over the years. I would love to share more with you in hopes of inspiring you to realize different ways that you may be able to give back to connections that are already established in your life.

Remember the pastor who ran the outreach initiative to feed underserviced members of my community? Well, he runs a Bible study group that I am so grateful to be a part of. As the name suggests, a Bible study group is a group of people who regularly get together to study the word of God, be it through reading the Bible, preaching or reciting intercessory prayers. My group meets every day for 30 minutes in the early morning, and we conduct our group over the telephone as our members reside in both Canada and in the United States. We all contribute by saying prayers or readings on a rotating basis. The pastor shares a sermon and always prompts us with things to reflect upon. Gathering in a Bible study group can offer so many opportunities to connect to things that are greater than you, and can be a place of growth and healing. I have had my own personal breakthroughs, all the while making new friends and supporting them and their break-throughs. It is a special and intimate circle of like-minded people that I have immense gratitude for.

Another way I plant good seeds in my life is by being a member of a mastermind alliance. These types of groups have existed since time immemorial! However, it was Napoleon Hill who defined a mastermind alliance and its potential in the book *Think and Grow Rich* in 1937. Since then, groups all over the world have formed with the intention of gathering in a structured environment and sharing in each other's wins and losses. My mastermind meets every Saturday morning for two hours. During that time, we each have an opportunity to share and dissect the advances or setbacks of our goals. We exchange ideas and outside perspectives for personal development. Each of us has our own strengths and expertise that we can bring to the group. That is why these groups are incredibly special and important. Our group is called the Eagles mastermind alliance and there is no investment to join. We have studied the book *Think and Grow Rich* and are currently studying *The Law of Success in Sixteen Lessons*. Both books were written by

Napoleon Hill. We are dedicated to each other's success and supporting one another as we strive for excellence. Not only have I found people to collaborate with on exciting ideas, I have also made lasting friendships.

In my professional life, I am very proud to have acquired three coaching designations. I received my Distinguished Toastmasters designation (the highest accolade bestowed on a Toastmasters member, obtained by only two percent of Toastmasters) through which I went on to mentor Toastmasters members. After obtaining my Distinguished Toastmasters designation, I ventured out and obtained a World Class Speaking Coach certificate from Craig Valentine, MBA (1999 World Class champion of Toastmasters). Toastmasters International is a worldwide non-profit educational organization that empowers individuals to become more effective communicators and leaders. Headquartered in Englewood, Colorado, USA, the organization's membership exceeds 357,000 people in more than 16,600 clubs in 143 countries. {Source: https://www.toastmasters.org}

Furthermore, I became a certified coach, speaker and trainer through The John Maxwell Company, which saw me being able to apply skills learned in order to teach French to international students on a private platform. Currently, I am also enrolled in a course to become a certified health and life coach with the aim to be certified in 2022. I love being able to help people level up their own skills in order to find new levels of success, no matter what they are trying to achieve. It feels like such an important aspect of why I am here. You can even see this through my writing this book! I want to see people succeed and thrive, and want to help in any way I can. I want to plant any good seeds, big or small, around me so that I may watch a beautiful garden of potential growth.

Of course, being of service to those around you in different ways is of great importance. However, you can never forget to also show up for yourself. You cannot just put your own well-being on the back burner and hope that you will be OK. You must learn to invest time and energy into your own self-care as well, so that you can keep showing up for your friends, family and community time and time again. Self-care needs to be a priority in your life. No excuses!

Chapter 7

Self-Care

*"I treat myself pretty good. I take lots of vacation,
I eat well, I take supplements, I do mercury detox,
I get plenty of sleep. I drink plenty of water
and I stay away from drama and stress."*
— Reba McEntire

Self-care can mean different things for different people. When it comes down to it, it does not matter what it really looks like, but adopting great self-care practices is absolutely essential when looking to beat cancer or help prevent it. Everything we have talked about to this point can be thought of as your foundation. The diet and everything we have spoken of are non-negotiables. Now upon that foundation you must build a self-care routine for yourself.

Perhaps you already have a self-care routine that you can just begin to incorporate once your foundation is in place. Fantastic! Start from there and also be open to new ideas. If building a self-care routine is new to you, do not worry. You can begin by exploring what feels good for you. Maybe there are already some things that pique your interest that you have always wanted to try. Or perhaps you have no idea where to start.

I will share with you some practices that I consider part of my self-care routine. Feel free to use them as jumping off points for your own exploration. Do not forget, self-care should feel good. It should not feel like a chore, or something you have to force yourself through. Sure, you may have to incorporate some discipline to show up to what you need to do. However, self-care should truly feel like the icing on the cake when it comes to adding to the routine you are already cultivating.

Exercise Regimen

I have always had some sort of exercise regime. Exercise makes me feel calm, healthy and relaxed. It also makes me sleep better. Because my mother was a registered nurse, from an early age both my parents always instilled in us the importance of exercise. I remember riding a bicycle from childhood into my teenage years, and even loving climbing the fruit trees that were in our backyard. My siblings and I also used to enjoy going swimming regularly. Being active was a natural part of my day-to-day life. My mother always used to say: "If you want to live long, exercise!" She is a testament of this statement because she went for walks until the ripe age of 85!

Prior to the Covid-19 pandemic, I participated in swimming and aquafit classes. (If you are not familiar with aquafit, it is where you essentially do aerobics in a swimming pool. It is very fun!) However, because of pandemic regulations the swimming pool closed in my condo and I had to find other ways to keep fit. Fitness had become such a part of my life that I needed to adapt in order to make sure it stayed part of my routine.

I decided to take on aerobics and brisk walking because they were cost-effective and fun to do. Aerobics can offer you so much with such little time commitment:

- Improves the efficiency of respiration
- Improves cardiovascular efficiency
- Strengthens your muscles
- Strengthens ligaments, tendons and bones
- Helps decrease anxiety and stress
- Helps decrease the risk of developing cancer, coronary artery disease, diabetes ... and more!

(Source: Ask an Expert: The Benefits of Aerobic Exercise. Providence Health & Services Oregon and Southwest Washington)

The benefits of exercise as part of a healthy way of living has been documented time and time again. However, if you are undergoing cancer treatment of any sort, it is especially important. The benefits are vast and may include:

- Reducing the onset of anxiety and depression
- Lowering the chance of having physical side effects such as fatigue, lymphedema (when legs and arms swell due to fluid retention), neuropathy (damage or dysfunction of nerves), osteoporosis and nausea
- Helping you remain as physically independent and mobile as possible
- Improving sleep. It is so important to get good sleep all the time but especially when undergoing treatment as it provides a chance for your body to heal.
- Helping reduce the risks of other cancers, and can act as preventative medicine
- It improves the survival rates for certain cancers such as breast and colo-rectal cancers
- and many more!

(Source: cancer.net/survivorship/healthy-living/erxercise-during-cancer-treatment)

Having an exercise regimen will improve your quality of life no matter what is going on. This is why it can be seen as an important part of your self-care routine. It can not only help you feel good in the moment, but is such an asset to your future health. Many people exercise not because of how they want to feel today, but because of how they want to feel in the days and the years to come! Find what works for you. It does not have to be a major commitment. The rule of thumb is to sweat about 20 minutes a day. Find what activities get you moving and find what time of day you feel best suits you. Perhaps you do something first thing in the morning and use it as an energy booster. Or perhaps you exercise in the afternoon as a pick me up. Explore and get creative. Create your own relationship to moving your body and this form of self-care.

Breast Care

When I had the tumuor in my right breast removed, the oncologist was so compassionate that he even apologized for leaving scars from the surgery. I told him that it was okay, because life is full of scars. As I have learned through this journey, our scars turn into stars, our disgrace into grace and our mess into a message.

My oncologist recommended I wear a comfortable sports bra for six weeks after my surgery. He recommended a sports bra specifically because they do not have any underwire built into them. I later found out from a friend of mine who is a nurse that underwire bras may cause breast cancer by blocking the drainage of lymph fluid from the bottom of the breast so it cannot get back into your body. Also, I quickly discovered that sports bras are more comfortable than conventional ones (especially when recovering from surgery). After the six weeks I continued to wear sports bras as much as possible as I found them extremely comfortable.

I find it interesting as the issue of wearing bras was brought up also with the homeopathic doctor I mentioned I had seen in 2014. After diagnosing that my right breast had not been functioning well, the homeopathic doctor advised that I should not wear a bra at home, or whenever I did not have to. I have taken all of this advice to heart. I no longer wear a bra, as much as possible. I am very conscious of this, as I now understand that it is not a good idea for my breast health. While bras are a part of life, it has become very clear to me that it is not healthy for the breasts themselves to always be wearing a bra. If you are a woman, I want you to take that to heart and stop wearing your bra as much as you can. Or perhaps wear a sports bra more as they are less restrictive for the tissues. I recollect as a teenager, when my mother returned home, she would always remove her bra... now I understand why!

There is an outdated idea that wearing a bra is thought to support the development of firm and well-formed breasts. However, new findings are proving this is not true. Studies have been continuously showing that bras do not prevent sagging or improve breast health in any way. They may actually be quite detrimental to the overall look of the breast and more importantly be detrimental in producing healthy breast tissue.

(Source: Benefits of going braless-Breast Enlargement Resource)

In terms of other ways, you can manage the health of your breast tissue is to actually give your breasts a massage regularly. There are some Registered Massage Therapists who offer breast massage. However, you can also do it yourself. I regularly massage my breasts, especially after the shower when I am applying moisturizer to my body. It is an excellent quick and easy way to add to your daily self-care. I recently learned from a registered nurse that the proper way to massage breasts is to rub each breast fifty times both clockwise and anti-clockwise to allow blood to circulate freely. I recall when I met with a homeopathic doctor, he also advised me to massage my breast in a similar fashion.

As part of my regular post cancer care, I have annual mammograms and ultrasounds on both my breasts. While this is necessary for me considering my health history, I recommend speaking to your health care provider about regular mammograms. This is an excellent part of preventative medicine. Part of the success of cancer diagnosis is early detection, and one way to detect a lump is when having a mammogram. I had earlier mentioned that mammograms are not hundred percent accurate. I caught the lump in my breast through self-examination. Because of my own ultrasounds, my oncologist was really able to gain insight as to how well my alternative treatments were working, and continue to keep my breasts cancer-free. It is imperative to get a sense of your breast health from the inside out so to speak.

I will reiterate the importance of breast self-examinations as the best way to find a lump when it is in its infancy. Again, if you are uncomfortable touching your own breasts, ask your partner to do it. If you do not have a partner, be willing to pay a massage therapist to do it for you. Incorporating this into your routine may save your life... it certainly saved mine!

Detoxification of Internal Organs

An important contributor to how I cured my breast cancer naturally was through the process of detoxing certain organs, specifically the liver, kidneys, and lymphatic systems. My holistic practitioner had me follow a certain protocol that I can share a part of with you to give you some insight. (Unfortunately, due to legal reasons I cannot fully disclose the names of all the products I used to support the detoxification process.) Focusing on detoxing your body is a personal act of self-care as it takes extra time, focus and effort in your day-to-day life. It is not necessarily an easy thing to experience. However, it is highly beneficial. I still have some detox protocols that I regularly engage in so that my body continues to stay as healthy as possible, and keep disease away.

The goal of detoxing was to remove built up toxins and excess mucus from my system so that my body could more effectively heal itself. The whole protocol lasted several days, and I was shocked as to how much junk and gunk came out of my body near the end of the time. It literally felt like I had an earthquake inside me and I actually ended up losing five pounds! I had friends who had similar experiences so I was not worried about the sort of effects it was having on my body. One of the most important things is to drink plenty of water in order to help the toxins flush properly and effectively from your body.

The first organ I specifically detoxed was my liver, as it is essential for cleaning your blood. The protocol my holistic practitioner provided me was pretty straightforward. I was to eat a breakfast and lunch that contained NO FATS whatsoever (no olive oil, no butter, no nuts), and stop all eating by 2pm.

I was then asked to follow this specific liver cleansing recipe of ingredients and timeline in order to effectively activate my liver.

Ingredients needed:

- 4 tablespoons of Epsom salt
- 2 red grapefruits
- 4 ounces (½ cup) extra virgin cold pressed olive oil
- 3 cups distilled water

6:00pm
- Mix 4 tablespoons of Epsom salt in 3 cups distilled water
- Drink ¾ Epsom salts mixture

8:00pm
- Drink ¾ cup Epsom salts mixture

9:30pm
- Squeeze the 2 red grapefruits by hand, remove pulp.
- Measure 2/3 cup of the juice and place into a bottle with a lid.
- Add to this 4-ounce extra virgin cold pressed olive oil and cover.
- Shake the contents the mixture vigorously to ensure ingredients are thoroughly mixed together

10:00pm
- Walk to your bedside and while standing, drink all of the olive oil/grapefruit mixture within 5 minutes.
- Lie on your back, head high on your pillow… stay in this position until you fall asleep. If you have to get up to go to the bathroom, go back

to bed right after. Lying on the back is important for the liver cleanse.

In the morning, it is important that you follow these steps:

6:30am
- Drink ¾ cup Epsom salt mixture

8:30am
- Drink ¾ cup Epsom salt mixture

10:30am
- Drink 1 cup of juice (any 100% juice, no sugar added, not from concentrate)

12:00pm
- Eat a piece of fruit (any variety, whole)

I continue to regularly practice different detoxification processes even now that I am cancer-free. I hold it as an important part of self-care practices. It makes me feel great and I think of it like a sort of tune up for my body.

Keeping a Gratitude Journal

The late Dr. Maya Angelou said:

"If you do not like something, change it.
If you cannot change it, change the way you think about it."

I like to keep this idea close as I navigate life. Especially when I am experiencing hardships. One of my mentors once advised me that in order to acquire anything of value, I must first show gratitude. This really struck me as I had not thought about my life like that before.

My personal reflection on gratitude is that we do not appreciate what we have until we have lost it. Connecting to gratitude is a powerful way that you can connect to your life.

If you are not familiar with exactly what a gratitude journal is, let me provide some insight and a jumping off point for you. You can use a diary or notebook of some sort. In it you will reflect on things you are grateful for. It can be any and all things... whatever is inspiring you that day! Perhaps you are grateful for the clean air to breathe or the clean running water you have access to. Perhaps you connect to things that are more personal to you. This is a personal gratitude journal just for you to both connect to the riches of your life in the moment as well as something that you may wish to refer back on as a reflective exercise.

Gratitude journals actually hold a lot of power and benefits that can add a lot of value to your life. A snapshot of these benefits include:

- Better psychological and physical health
- Experiencing more empathy and less aggressive feelings towards others
- Greater mental strength
- Better sleep
- Become more resilient in your life
- Experience more experience creativity
- ...and more!

(Source: Lauren Jessen, The Benefits of a Gratitude Journal)

Listen to Relaxing Music

Music is often referred to as an international language. It is a language without words, but is communication through sound! When I was deep in the process of healing my cancer, my holistic doctor advised me to avoid placing myself in any stressful situations. This is due to the fact that one of the causes of cancer is chronic stress. So, I had to be very mindful of what environments I was creating around myself.

I turned to music to help create more relaxing healing spaces in my life. Because of not wanting to induce stress I was very particular of the music I chose. For me, classical and gospel music make me feel relaxed and at ease. Some of my favourite classical pieces include Water Music by Handel, and anything that is piano based. If you are not familiar with gospel music, it is a genre of Christian music that I personally find very soothing.

What kind of music makes you feel calmer and more grounded? It is fun to experiment and discover what makes you feel good. You can use the music that you choose to shift you into a calmer state when you need it. You can play it at specific times of your day, or perhaps use it as a tool to use when you feel your stress levels rising. However you use it, be open to connecting to the power of music as a way to help you heal and keep you healthy.

Have a Laugh!

I am sure you have heard the old adage "Laughter is the best medicine!" Laughter has extraordinary healing properties for the body. I once read about a man who after a long battle of cancer was given only a few months to live. He decided to watch comedy shows all day long in order to connect with laughter and bring more joy into what was supposed to be darker days. I am not sure really how it happened, but the man did not die from his illness and survived his diagnosis.

There are incredible noted health benefits of laughter:

- It fortifies your immune system
- It helps you feel less pain (both physically and emotionally)

- It can increase blood flow through the body, most specifically to the heart
- It is shown to reduce inflammation
- It can help reduce anxiety and boost your mood in a more positive way
- Laughter helps you make it through tough times
- …. and much more!

(Source: "20 Crazy Health Benefits of Laughter-No Joke" Tehrene Firman, July 26, 2018)

I had to figure out a way to bring more laughter into my life. The first thing I did was subscribe to an email service that sent a joke each day to my inbox. What a delight it is to receive a joke in my inbox every morning! It gives me something to smile about before I have to think about the more serious things in my life.

I also volunteered for the role of "Joke Master" during my time with Toastmasters. As I previously mentioned, Toastmasters International is an international association where people enroll to improve on their communication, leadership and presentation skills.

While in Toastmasters there are different club roles that one may take on, with one of them being the "Joke Master" or humorist of your club. Essentially I usually volunteered to share jokes in an effort to lighten the mood of meetings. Cracking jokes certainly made me feel less stress and anxiety, and I could clearly see how it made other members feel at ease. I really enjoyed my time in that position!

I hope that you are inspired to dive deeper into your own self-care practices. If up until this point in your life you have not really thought about it, I hope that you move forward and find ways to make self-care part of your daily life.

Beyond self-care there is another layer of taking care of yourself and continuing to build upon that foundation that we spoke of. Have you ever thought about ways that you can "fertilize" your body with more energy and life force? I want to talk about it a bit deeper so that you may gain insight as to how you can apply these incredible practices yourself and take good care.

Chapter 8

"Fertilize" Your Body

"A healthy lifestyle includes exercise, nutrition, healthy sleep patterns and a healthy group of friends."
— Sophie Grégoire Trudeau

8

I love that quote because it always reminds me that there is an argument for the simple things. This next layer of your wellness journey goes beyond self-care. It is all about finding things in addition to everything we have talked about in order to create a well "fertilized" body that can continue to support your growth and the great health you have found. Your journey to conquering cancer or preventing it is multifaceted. I want to share some things I feel are more subtle and were added to my routine once I had established the foundation of my protocols. You can take these for your own, or perhaps they will inspire you to get curious about your own unique ways of fertilizing your own body. Find what works for you!

Soak Up the Sun

It is of utmost importance to get enough sun. Sunshine triggers production of Vitamin D, which is an essential nutrient needed in the body. (I spoke about this in Chapter 4.) However, did you know that sitting in the sunshine can also help you with so much more? Think about it. I am sure that there are times where you have naturally craved feeling the sun on your skin or face. Perhaps it was after a long winter (if in the northern hemisphere). Perhaps after a stretch of rainy days.

As humans, we are naturally attracted to the sunshine! Its health benefits really knows no bounds:

- It boosts your mood
- Reduces stress and pain associated with surgery
- Builds the immune system
- It can reduce cancer risks (because of the Vitamin D that it will naturally produce in your body)
- Naturally kills bad bacteria
- and more!

(Source: Hamilton Recruitment: Caribbean & Bermuda Jobs)

How do you usually get some sunshine? I will make an effort to sit out on my balcony or go for a walk with the goal to simply soak up the sun. I have also got into the habit of parking a bit further from entrances when I am out and about so that I may get some sun while walking to the door of a shop or business. These are easy ways to incorporate more sun into your schedule while you go about your daily business.

When I was first discussing this with my holistic health practitioner, she brought up the fact that dark skinned people (as I am) need more sunshine than caucasian individuals. This is because it takes longer for dark skinned people to manufacture and synthesize the sun into Vitamin D. On top of this I have to be extra mindful because I live in Canada, so the amount of direct sun I can actually obtain is quite less compared to when living in tropical countries.

When you commit to spending time in the sun, you not only greatly affect your physical health but you fertilize great things for all aspects of you. Getting sun is multidimensional in its healing properties.

Drinking My "Daily Concoction"

As discussed in Chapter 3, garlic and lemons both have great nutritional value. Another way that I boost my intake of these potent, healing foods is to drink 1.5 ounces of a blend of organic garlic and organic lemon. My health practitioner recommended this sort of "health shot" as a way to increase my intake of the amazing benefits of the garlic and lemon combined. Of course, this concoction is not for the faint of heart! The smell and taste are quite pungent and if you are not used to it, it may take some time to adapt. However, as with anything new, habit or routine, you certainly do get used to it! I have actually come to enjoy this part of my daily routine as I can clearly connect to the amazing healing properties that I am putting in my body to my high level of physical health.

Why garlic and lemon together? Well, firstly the taste is actually quite nice. I am sure you may think of a few dishes where garlic and lemon are used to create some incredible tasting food. So, it can be seen as a flavor shot. We widely covered the health benefits of garlic. In addition to things mentioned, the sulphureous compounds in garlic are where the cancer fighting magic lies. These particular compounds have been studied for their ability to inhibit cancerous cells and block tumors by slowing DNA replication. Incredible! Adding the power of lemon on top of that really takes it to the next level. Not only does lemon have numerous health benefits ranging from managing hypertension to aiding in weight loss, it has been found to help kill cancer cells. *(Source: The Benefits and Uses for Lemon Juice for Cancer by Dr Maria. Health and Wellness, May 5, 2018)* According to a study published in 2016 on nutrients, lemons have anticancer benefits for prostate, breast, stomach, liver, cervix, pancreas and colon cancer cells. It is important to note that these findings are from controlled studies on cancer cells in a lab.

(Source: Lemons and cancer: Are they protective? Livestrong.com)

Drinking this shot of garlic and lemon every day makes me feel revitalized and connected to my physical health. It is an idea not for everyone, but I had to share it as it makes me feel incredible. It certainly was a game changer.

Enjoying Fresh Fruit and Vegetable Smoothies

A fantastic way to ensure you are getting enough of the various fruits and vegetables that are important to eat when looking to prevent or fight cancer is to drink them! Smoothies are drinks made with blended fruits and vegetables, and a fantastic way to incorporate more powerful, raw foods into your diet.

I love all smoothie flavors and really do not have a favourite one. I did not think to drink them before my holistic practitioner recommended them because of their health benefits. Now I usually enjoy them on weekends for breakfast when I am not practicing intermittent fasting. I noticed that when I started drinking smoothies, they gave me a heightened sense of well-being! I'm guessing it is from all the incredible ingredients packed into one drink!

The benefits of drinking fresh smoothies are plentiful:

- Because of the high-water content in the fruits and vegetables, they can help prevent dehydration
- Controls mood swings and helps fight depression
- They are a high dose of good fiber
- Assists in detoxing the body
- May balance hormonal functioning
- A great source of antioxidants which can help keep in check the growth of free radicals and other cancer-causing agents

- Depending on ingredients, will reduce the chance of cancers (example broccoli and cauliflower are fantastic cancer fighting ingredients you can easily add to your smoothies)
- ... and more!

(Source: https://easyhealthysmoothie.com)

Incorporating smoothies into my routine is such a lovely ritual for me. Again, I know that I am taking the time to do something good for my body. But it goes beyond just the ingredients. Making and drinking smoothies has become a ritual that not only nourishes my body but also my mind. It asks me to take a break in my day and do something good for myself.

Hydrate! Hydrate! Hydrate!

When I began my cancer fighting journey, I had been told by several doctors that I was not drinking enough water. I admit, drinking enough water and staying hydrated was not really on my radar when it came to thinking about my health. But since I began the process of detoxing my internal organs and switching my focus to living a life where I am in good health, drinking enough water has certainly become a priority. You may have the same struggle when it comes to drinking enough water, but once you change a few habits it is not as hard as you think.

Upon waking in the morning, the first thing I do is drink a glass of water. I usually keep a glass of water on my night stand in case I feel thirsty during the night. If I do not drink it then, it is already waiting for me when I wake up! I make an effort to drink a glass of water around my meals as opposed to with my food. I find that is more effective in actually hydrating me. So, I will tend to drink a glass of water 30 minutes before eating, then also wait until 30 minutes after to have a glass.

Another new habit that I now have is keeping a bottle of water in my purse at all times. It is then readily available to sip on when I am driving somewhere, or when I am out and about running errands. It is really important to have water immediately available when you are thirsty. Essentially always keep some water nearby and begin noticing when you are thirsty, or just get into the habit of always sipping your water. It will become something that you no longer have to think about.

A simple way I learned to determine if I am drinking enough water and staying hydrated throughout my day is to examine my urine when I go to the washroom. This is one of the simplest ways of knowing if you need to be drinking more water, even if you are not necessarily thirsty. If the color of your urine is dark yellow, this is an indication of being dehydrated. If it is pale yellow in color, then you are drinking enough water. This is a quick and easy way to take stock of your hydration level. If you wish to have more of an actual calculation, it is easy to predetermine the ideal amount of water you should be drinking in a day. Take your weight in pounds and divide it into two, and that is the number of ounces of water you should be consuming in a day. For example, if you weigh 150 pounds, half of that is 75, so your daily intake of water with that weight would be 75 ounces of water.

The quality of the water you are drinking is important. I always boil my water first and then use a standard filter. I also keep my water in a vessel at room temperature. I find my teeth are too sensitive to drink cold things. (Sometimes I will even add some lemon slices, flaxseed or apple cider vinegar to make my water more flavorful!) However, some also feel that drinking cold water can be detrimental to your health. I remember when I lived in Asia, I noticed no one drank cold beverages with any of their meals. They instead chose hot soup or tea. Of course, this is very different from standard North American practices. People there would tell me that illnesses could be cured by drinking hot beverages. They also expressed that they believed people in the western countries suffered from clogged arteries because they ate hot food with cold water... What an interesting perspective!

When I am hydrated, I feel good. I have learned that staying hydrated really keeps my head clear, and I am able to stay motivated and focused. I cannot believe that it was not until my health failed that I really paid attention to my water intake. If you already drink enough water, good for you! If not, I urge you to start today to create this new habit.

Find Health Specialists to Work With

You cannot do it alone. No matter how hard you try in order to gain optimal health I think it is really important to find different health practitioners that you want to engage with to make your ultimate health team. After my cancer diagnosis, it became essential to visit my holistic health practitioner once a month or every other month in order to keep up with the different protocols that were necessary as I opted out of chemotherapy treatment. It was great to touch base with someone who I knew wanted to help me and had my best interest at heart. I learned so much from her and knew I could count on her support through that difficult time.

If you find you have to manage anything health wise, be it acute or chronic, minor or serious, there are specialists in every single field ready to help you. I feel this is an important part of your commitment to "fertilize" your body well so that you may grow your potential. There are no limits to what this can look like in your life. However, you cannot go it alone. Trust me. Find the support you need and then watch yourself grow and succeed in whatever you put your mind to! I remain forever grateful to my holistic doctor for helping me conquer my breast cancer, and teaching me how to continue supporting my health in order to live cancer-free.

I hope that you see the different ways in which you may help yourself to create a fertile life in which you may thrive and reach your health goals. Never forget that every single thing you commit to can and will help you in the long run.

I have briefly touched upon the spiritual aspect of healing in previous chapters. However, it is now time to do a deeper dive. I want to share with you how keeping the faith and having hope played essential roles in my cancer journey.

Chapter 9

The Power of Faith and Hope

*"Be faithful in small things because
it is in them that your strength lies."*
— Mother Teresa

9

An important aspect of my healing journey without having to use chemotherapy was committing to have a stronger, more vertical fellowship with God. I had always been a faithful person but when I was faced with the news of my cancer diagnosis, I had to take a step back and start really examining what was important to me. The way I had been living my life up until that point was in line with my faith but I knew that if I made a new commitment my healing journey would be infused with more light and hope.

The Bible states: "But Jesus looked at them and said, "With man this is impossible, but with God all things are possible." {Matthew 19:26} Let me show you how I developed a stronger relationship with God and how it brought much inspiration to my life.

Daily Morning Devotionals

What if you started your day by taking a few minutes to sit and connect with something that is greater than yourself? This is where daily devotionals can help. Daily devotionals are Christian religious publications that provide specific spiritual readings for each calendar day. They are either published as a monthly or yearly collection.

First and foremost, when I wake up the first thing, I say to start off my day is: "Good morning Holy Spirit, thank you for waking me up from sleep!"

I never want to take for granted the fact that I actually woke up and I am alive to live another day. I then move to read the devotional. I open up the page that corresponds to the date and take some time to read what is offered. The formats are reflections or short prayers, and have a corresponding biblical reference. There is always a great uplifting title that will give you an idea of the theme of the day. Here are some examples:

- Your Root is Growing Strong, Never Quit Now!
- The Secret of Shutting the Door
- There is a Minstrel in You!
- Faith-Building Memories
- I am an Eagle and Not a Grasshopper
- The Power of Prayer
- and many more.....

(Source: Our Daily Manna: A Daily Devotional Booklet for Champions July to September 2021)

Devotionals are highly beneficial to your life. By offering God your devotion, you may receive guidance in return. You get to not only know yourself better, but also develop a stronger relationship with Jesus, as well as the Holy Spirit. In our crazy, fast-paced world it presents an opportunity to sit still. It is also a fantastic way to bring your family and loved ones together and create a deeper personal relationship with them. All in all, devotionals are a great way to help manage stress, which you certainly know is necessary to lead a healthier life. *(Source: Call to Glory, an independent, fundamental Baptist, king James Devotional)*

I find devotionals very positive, thought-provoking and uplifting. After taking time to read them, I feel ready to tackle my day with gusto! Devotionals help strengthen all parts of me: spiritually, physically and mentally. This in turn no doubt helps strengthen my immune system and helps prevent illness.

Listen to Gospel and Classical Music

As I previously mentioned, I love lifting my spirits by listening to gospel and classical music. I have always had an appreciation for classical music since I was younger. (I wish I never gave up learning to play the piano!) These genres of music keep me feeling relaxed and grounded.

Gospel music specifically is a type of Christian music that is very devotional to God, Jesus and the Holy Spirit. This music promotes faith and inspires the soul. I will literally listen to it throughout my whole day: when I am in the shower, taking a walk, in the car... anywhere! It helps me remember the more important things in life.

Gospel music has been found to give people a sense of purpose (source: Abbey Cheche, Arts and Entertainment, April 18, 2018) When you are in the middle of healing yourself from cancer or managing any other health issues, it is essential to have a sense of something bigger and better coming your way. It can instill a sense of hope for the days ahead.

Classical music has always been seen as a wonderful tool to use in people's healing processes. Whether it be managing pain, improving sleep or enhanced mental alertness, this type of music can be great to reach for in the middle of a healing journey or to keep disease at bay. *(Source: Shari Mathias, Parker Symphony Orchestra)*

As I went through my own healing journey, both gospel and classical music helped me relax and at times take me away to a different place; a place where I was very healthy and felt incredible. Again, these music genres were able to help me keep my faith, even on darker days. It helped me remain grounded and focused on the brighter days ahead.

Daily Intercessory Prayer

If you are not familiar with it, intercessory prayer is praying on behalf of others or for the needs of others. It is a different way of connecting to praying to God as your prayers are focused on others. For example, the week's schedule for my group may look like this:

- Monday we pray for each other's family
- Tuesday we pray for our pastors
- Wednesday we pray for government leaders
- Thursday we pray for students
- Friday we pray for business owners
- Saturday we pray for teachers

As I mentioned in Chapter 6, I feel blessed to be part of a prayer and Bible study group that meets daily. We have all committed to be on the telephone from 6-6:30am (or until 7am Saturday). We have a schedule where we consciously pray for people within the group. We are seven members and two of the same members are scheduled to pray on Mondays and Wednesdays; two others are scheduled to pray on Tuesdays and Thursdays. Two are scheduled to lead prayers on Thursdays; two others on Fridays and two on Saturdays. We have Sunday off to sleep in. The pastor will also have a topic for each day, for which he will offer his own reflection on as well as scriptures from the Bible. Topics may include such things as anger, healing, righteousness, grace, hope, and kindness.

I pray constantly and feel prayer can offer so much to the individual:

- A better sense of self
- Good for your heart
- Increases life span
- Improves attitude
- Gain forgiveness
- Relieves stress

- Maintain a positive outlook on life
- Recovery: "After a situation leaves you emotionally or physically distraught, recovery is a timely process. Prayer serves as a way to deal with the aftermath and keep one's faith. Your body and mind are focused solely on healing while prayer keeps you centered and hopeful."

(Source: Top 10 Health Benefits of Praying by Health Fitness Revolution, May 21, 2015)

My prayer group offered me their own prayers on a daily basis, and this was part of the reason I healed.

Reading From the Bible Daily

If you want to boost your joy and increase your overall awareness, reading from the Bible daily can be a powerful tool. I mentioned that, as part of my prayer group, we read scripture daily. I love when it is my turn to share the powerful words of God with my friends. Starting the day this way always gives me a great boost of inspiration and propels me forward to have a productive day.

Reading the Bible is a rich and fulfilling experience. It pleases God when you connect to these powerful words and brings you closer to Divinity. Doesn't that sound like a nice place to be?

Sit in a "Thinking" Chair

I am sure it is becoming clear that I have a regular morning routine that helps me connect to God and my faith. Another lovely thing I do each morning is take some time to sit in my Thinking Chair. I learned this exercise from one of my mentors years ago.

As part of your morning devotional time, you simply sit and think. Make sure the chair is comfortable. Perhaps it is in a nice area of your home. You simply take the time to sit, be quiet and think. It is a personal exercise that you can make your own. During my time in my Thinking Chair, I like to focus on how I can better all the facets of my life: spiritual, financial, physical, social, emotional and mental. Sometimes I walk away just having enjoyed connecting with my thoughts. Sometimes I walk away with a great idea or an answer to a problem that needs to be solved. In any regard, it is never wasted time.

A big part of improving my life is also how I may be of service to others. Motivational speaker Zig Ziglar said:

"If you help enough people get what they want, you will get what you want."

I take this to heart, and bring a lot of focus to being of benefit to others. It was especially helpful during the time while I was fighting my breast cancer. It helped me take focus from myself and place it on others, which felt good. It reminded me that there was more to my life than just my cancer journey.

I had lots of amazing moments in my Thinking Chair, and would never miss my session. Even when I am pressed for time, I will still always take at least a few minutes to just stop, and think.

When I commit to beginning each day with my morning devotion, it gives me the faith and hope to conquer all adversities I may face now and in the future. While I was managing my cancer recovery it was absolutely necessary to deepen my connection to God in any way I could. Having faith in a higher power helped me become steadfast, and directly played a part in conquering my breast cancer, no doubt!

I also had an incredible support circle of friends and family praying for me, and keeping the faith that I would come through the other side.

Even my own pastor, upon finding out about my diagnosis, declared that I would not die, and would live to share my testimony. (And here I am writing this book!)

Keeping hope alive within yourself and surrounding yourself with people who believe in you is powerful. There are studies out there which state that those who were optimistic during their illnesses got better faster than those who were negative:

"For decades, many researchers thought the boost in immunity was as a result of the fact that optimistic people were more likely to take care of their health. But more recent studies have shown that a hopeful outlook is actually what influences immunity. Looking on the bright side makes you less likely to get a cold or infection because optimism keeps your immune system performing at its peak." *(Source: 7 Ways to heal your body by using the power of your mind, backed by science by Amy Morin)* Remaining hopeful and positive was part of what saved me.

Because of my battle with breast cancer, my life changed for the better. Some of these changes were big and some were subtle. Let me share with you what my life looked like and felt like after I was diagnosed and cured. I am forever changed and would never trade my experience for anything.

Chapter 10

My Life After Breast Cancer

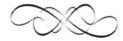

"A man's legacy is determined by how the story ends."
— Leonardo DiCaprio

10

Because of my breast cancer journey, my life certainly changed dramatically. Now that I am back to full health after beating the cancer naturally, I can clearly see what a blessing in disguise that journey was. My life is forever changed for the better and I will forever be grateful for what I have learned.

I want to share with you some reflections on how I feel now, the changes I experienced and invite you to reflect on how you may continue to grow and expand your own life. Even if you are going through your own struggles or challenges, life has so much to offer you in return for you trying new things or showing up more than ever before.

Give More, Appreciate Life More

As I mentioned before, while I was undergoing my recovery to better health, I was invited to help feed the homeless and less privileged every Sunday with some members from my Bible study group. My perspective on how I interact with my community changed dramatically during that time. I could clearly feel that the more I was willing to give, the more I appreciated all the goodness in my own life.

It is a strong team of five people and we manage to feed about 50-80 homeless people every Sunday in downtown Toronto. I find it distressing that I live in a rich country such as Canada and there are people who do not have food to eat. I have met many of these less fortunate people and am grateful, as I doubt I would have crossed paths with them otherwise.

Creating a relationship with this community through our efforts every Sunday makes me feel like I am giving back in some small way. In turn, it makes my own life feel even more rich and fulfilling.

Connect to Even More Gratitude

As I mentioned before, having an attitude of gratitude is an essential part of a healing journey. It keeps you connected to the bigger picture. I continue to keep a gratitude journal to this day. I take some time to write in it every night before I go to bed. It always makes me feel calm and less stressed before I close my eyes for the night. Keeping up with my gratitude practices has also allowed me to further learn a lot about myself, and heightens my self-awareness. I also love having a record of reflections that I can refer back to when I need a solid reminder of all the good in my life.

I noticed that after incorporating a conscious gratitude practice I have a far greater appreciation for the finer things in life. As well, I can easily see more opportunities to share my riches when good things come into my life. Perspective is everything when it comes to being grateful for what you have.

Self-Improvement

I have always been a curious person and committed to growth. However, I found that during my cancer journey I began to put extra focus on my life outside of work and began seeing my life with a broader lens. The ways I engage with my own self-improvement expanded and still are with me today. Let me briefly share with you some highlights in hope that it may inspire you to keep growing and committing to something more in your life.

Read More Books

One of my mentors always said "Readers are leaders." After I conquered my breast cancer, I found that I began reading a lot more than usual. Of course, we were all at home more because of the pandemic. However, I could not get enough of reading self-development books and became fascinated as to how I could best use this life that had been gifted to me. (This also led to attending more online classes and seminars, all with focuses on self-improvement.) Making reading a part of your everyday life is highly beneficial for your overall health. Beyond improving your brain connectivity and preventing cognitive decline, reading has been shown to lower your heart rate and blood pressure and help fight depression (source: Rebecca Joy Stanborough, MFA October 15, 2019)

If you already do not have a strong relationship with reading, I urge you to find the time and make it happen. You will notice a difference in your life.

Take Online Courses

As I mentioned above, I found myself taking more online courses. Of course, during the pandemic everything moved to virtual platforms. But this was such a gift! Suddenly I could take classes and courses that were not available to me before they went online. Some were free and some I definitely made the financial investment in when I felt it to be of value. To be honest, I really enjoyed taking classes online in the comfort of my own home. It makes me feel less stressed and more comfortable.

Eating Well

When I began changing my eating habits during my journey to conquer cancer, my holistic doctor always reminded me to "Let food be thy medicine and let medicine be thy food." (Source: Hippocrates, Greek Physician.) By this adage, Hippocrates was emphasizing the importance of nutrition to prevent or cure disease. Learning more about how food affected my health caused me to make many changes to my diet, many of which I still practice today. Sometimes it can be tricky in my personal life as I have to decline social invitations at times. However, I would never exchange the way I now feel for anything.

Managing Stress

In our modern world, there is no way to escape stress altogether. However, over the course of my healing journey it became very clear to me the importance of managing stress in your life and managing it well.

As I mentioned at the beginning of the book, one of the possible causes of cancer is stress. This is because of the effects of stress on the body. At the time of publishing this book I am studying to become a certified health and life coach and, during my studies, the ways in which stress negatively affects the body has come up numerous times.

The list is quite extensive, but let me share a few highlights with you:

- Increases inflammation in the body which can be the basis for many diseases
- Causes a lowering of levels in growth hormones which are essentially healing, rebuilding and growing all tissues in the body
- Increases resistance to insulin, resulting in diabetes, heart disease and weight gain
- Decreases nutrient absorption and increase nutrient excretion

- Decreases sex hormones, resulting in a decrease in muscle mass or lower sex drive

(Source: The Effects of Stress on the Body, Health Coach Institute)

I could go on. I am sure this snapshot gives you a sense of how stress infiltrates all systems in our body and causes great harm.

In order to manage stress, there are many ways you can approach it, and many activities you can do. The following are what works very well for me, that I include regularly in my days in order to keep my stress in check.

Take Naps - Every day I take time for a "siesta" which is an afternoon nap. I aim for thirty minutes; however, sometimes that changes depending on my schedule for the day. These days I mainly work from home so fitting in a nap is much easier. Taking time every day for major relaxation, be it a nap or otherwise, is very strengthening for your immune system. There are some companies such as Google which have sleeping pods that they encourage their employees to use, and take twenty minute power naps in order to stay rejuvenated and energized.

Daily Walk - Every day I go for a brisk walk. If I can, I will try to get it in during the morning to give myself an energetic boost. I make an effort to keep a brisk pace and also swing my arms in order to get my heart rate up. My daily walk lightens my mood and feels energizing! It gives me a more positive outlook on my day. I really notice a difference in my mind and body when I cannot fit it in.

Breathe Deeply - Breathing deeply is another way I bring things back into focus, so to speak. It helps me get present and makes my mind feel more clear and at ease. There is a technique that I regularly use, especially if I am feeling a bit higher level of stress than usual. It is called the box breathing method or square breathing. What you do is consciously bring your breath into four parts. You can try it right now with me. Inhale deeply into your belly for four counts. Gently hold the breath for four counts. Slowly exhale the breath for four counts and hold the breath out for four counts. Continue this breath cycle for as long as is required. It is an incredible tool that can make your mind feel more centered very quickly.

Get a Massage - I began getting regular massages after my lumpectomy that I received right after my cancer diagnosis. I really noticed the positive effects in my life so I have chosen to keep massages as a part of my regular routine. They help me feel more rejuvenated and almost like a new person! It is very powerful how much getting a massage can shift your perspective and outlook.

Comedies, Movies and Sermons

After healing from this dreadful disease, I now will always make time to have a laugh, watch a film and connect with God. I have mentioned all of the above during the course of the book. But I am highlighting them one more time because this is how important they still are to me.

I love watching comedy shows, from television series to stand up specials. They never cease to just make me feel better when I need a "pick me up." I love that I can turn on my television and something can offer the medicine of laughter so quickly to me. The same with watching a movie. Movies are a chance to escape your own life for a while, but I always come away feeling like I learned something about humans or myself. Storytelling in the form of a film is a very powerful way to connect to things that are outside of your world. In addition to Hollywood films, I also love watching Bollywood and Nollywood.

In terms of engaging with sermons, we are so lucky now as there are many sermons available online and on television. I can either just tune in and be reminded of God's powerful words and teachings, or I can specifically seek out a sermon that I need to hear. They always help me remain present in my own life and connect deeply to what really matters.

My life after conquering cancer feels full and exciting. I feel grateful that I went through my experience. No matter how hard challenges seemed at the time, I can now see how it was all worth it. Today, I feel like a more whole person, and all the lessons I learned were invaluable.

This journey has been so inspiring in fact, that I decided to enroll and become a certified health and life coach. Even beginning to write this book solidified for me that I want to continue to help people in their own health the best I can. Let us all remember that health is wealth. There is always light at the end of the tunnel!

Chapter 11

Transforming Into a Certified Health and Life Coach

*"When you focus on your health,
you awaken your creativity. By creativity,
I don't mean painting or drawing,
I mean the ability to conceive your life
exactly the way you most want it."*
— Stacey Morgenstern, Founder at Health Coach Institute

*"In order to master aliveness -- in life and in business --
we must let go of the habit of being stopped."*
— Carey Peters, Founder at Health Coach Institute

11

Throughout my life I have had my fair share of health concerns. I have managed and overcome several major health issues including anemia, hypertension, uterine fibroids and then most recently breast cancer. After coming through the other side, my passion for health and wellness is stronger than it has ever been! It became clear to me that I wanted to share this passion with you, not only through this book but also through starting a new chapter in my life to become a certified health and life coach.

My aim as a health and life coach is to make an impact and help transform people's lives through 20% teaching then 80% transformation. A health and life coach can be many things to different people, depending on one's goals and what is needed. We are advocates for change, transformation and healthy habits. Imagine having a teacher who can assist you in your transformation as well as act as an accountability partner to keep you on track while you are committing to creating change? This is why I am training to be one. I want to be part of people's transformation. I believe in the possibility of anyone creating changes for the better in their lives. If I can do it, so can you!

I hope you enjoyed reading about my healing journey and how I conquered breast cancer without the use of chemotherapy. What an incredible journey it has been and continues to be! Who would have thought that my life would change so drastically for the better as I faced one of the most difficult challenges I hope I will ever face?

If you leave this time together with anything I hope you never forget that:

HEALTH IS WEALTH!

Francisca is available for speaking engagements.
If you are interested in an appearance at your business, event, congregation or conference, please send an email to:

breastcancerconquerednow@gmail.com

Acknowledgements

A book is never accomplished alone! There is a score of people who knowingly or unknowingly contributed to the successful germination, development and completion of this book.

I am especially grateful to Dr. Debra Williams ND, Lifestyle Educator, Medical Missionary and Health Director in Jamaica, whose story of curing her breast cancer without chemotherapy inspired and motivated me to believe it was possible. Thank you for giving me permission to quote your name within chapters in my book.

Special thanks to my publisher Raymond Aaron and his team, the Raymond Aaron Group, for their relentless editing and publication of this book. Without their professionalism and excellence, this book would not have been shared with the world.

My heartfelt appreciation is extended to Pastors Solomon and Constance Wunibee of Wisdom Embassy Church, Toronto, who prayed and laid hands on me declaring that I would be cancer-free and that I would have a testimony.

I deeply appreciate the wisdom of my healthcare providers: my oncologist, family doctor, dietician and holistic practitioner. (Their names are not mentioned due to patient/doctor privacy and confidentiality.) You made an amazing healthcare team through such a difficult time.

Thank you very much for the advice I received from a lawyer at Legal Shield concerning the legal aspects of my book.

I would like to acknowledge the support and encouragement from the active members of my weekly group, Eagles Mastermind Alliance: Trudy Bak, Jeff Ginsbarg, Leah Xing, Wanda Zayachkowski, Karolina Undak, Sherman Daley, Bob Doepel, and John Demaniuk.

Many thanks to those who had so much confidence in me that they pre-ordered my book before the release date, including Trudy Bak, Lessie Rodriguez and my cousins Andrea Turner and Heather Gobern.

My heartfelt appreciation is extended to the following people who have given me stellar testimonials: Pastor Lumembo Tshiswaka, Jeffrey Ginsbarg, Leah Xing, Thomas Eyambe, Wilma David, Eric Lofholm, Trudy Bak, Hailey Patry. You continue to inspire me each day.

To Carey Peters and Stacey Morgenstern, founders and primary teachers of Health Coach Institute (where I am pursuing certification to become a health and life coach). Thank you for your insight and mastery of several health-related topics.

Finally, I am grateful to the Almighty for having healed me, keeping me alive and giving me the courage, fortitude and wisdom to share my story!

About the Author

Francisca Epale is the award-winning author of *The Naked Educator: How to Survive in the Middle Kingdom (2016)* and *The Naked Educator: Secrets to Surviving in China as an Expatriate, second edition. (2018).*

She has taught English as a second language and French in the United States of America, Canada and China for more than 20 years, from the public school system to post-secondary levels. Francisca proudly holds a Bachelor of Arts in French from Edinboro University Edinboro, PA, USA and a Master of Arts in Teaching French as a Foreign Language from Mankato State University (now Minnesota State University), Mankato, MN, USA.

Her certificates to teach English include: TESL Ontario from (CCLCS) Canadian Centre for Language and Cultural Studies; TESL Canada from Hansa Language Centre and TESOL from Global TESOL College (all based in Toronto, Ontario, Canada.) Francisca is also an accredited community French interpreter in Ontario, Canada.

In addition to her own publications, Francisca is also a contributing author and international bestselling author of *365 Empowering Stories: Stories and Poems That Will Inspire And Empower You And Bring More Laughter, Joy And Love To Your life! (2019).* Her contribution entitled *My Journey: The Seven Amazing Steps that Shrunk My Uterine Fibroids* was celebrated and well received.

Francisca has acquired her Distinguished Toastmasters Designation (DTM), the highest award bestowed on a Toastmasters member (with only 2% of members ever attaining this coveted award!). In addition to this great accolade, Francisca is also a certified World Class Speaking coach through Craig Valentine, MBA (1999 World Champion of Toastmasters International) and a certified independent John Maxwell coach, speaker and trainer.

Francisca is a perpetual learner, and because of her passion to coach, empower and inspire people about her breast cancer journey, she is currently studying to become a certified Health and Life Coach through the Health Coach Institute, USA. (Expected graduation is 2022.)

During her leisure time, Francisca enjoys reading, writing books, watching movies, brisk walking, jogging and aerobics. Francisca Epale is available to deliver keynote presentations and coaching for individuals or groups. For rates and availability, please contact: breastcancerconquerednow@gmail.com.